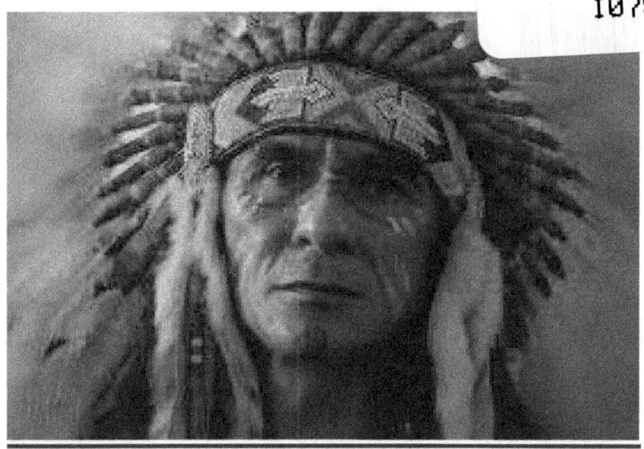

The Essiac Story

How an ancient Native American herbal remedy has helped modern mankind

By Larry Thomas

Table of Contents

Author's note:

In 1990 a well-known and very successful Los Angeles chiropractor named Gary Glum began to expound on the amazing healing qualities of an ancient indian herbal remedy from Canada. Magazine articles were written about it, and the Internet had good coverage of his presentations.

I was given a sample of the herbal tea. I gave it to a friend of mine who was very sick with lupus. My friend made a quick and dramatic comeback. This really got my attention.

Thus began my investigations into this herbal remedy that was named Essiac Tea. It also led me down the rabbit hole into the wonderful and sometimes mysterious world of alternative medicine. My life has been altered for the better by this experience, especially when I used the tea to cure myself of cancer in 2000.

So I have written this book to tell you the story of Essiac tea. May it help you, as it helped me!!

Foreword

For years now I have been interested in alternative cures for debilitating diseases which seem to threaten all of us, such as cancer, AIDS, multiple sclerosis, lupus, chronic fatigues, Alzheimer's, etc. In the course of pursuing this interest, I was enthusiastic about some treatment methods that appeared successful. However, this enthusiasm was nothing compared to the enthusiasm and excitement I felt when I discovered the story of Rene Caisse's herbal remedy that she called Essiac.

I believe that you will find this story very informative and interesting. The story of the development of Essiac, the struggle to get this knowledge out to the public, and the information available about the documented cases of thousands of persons being cured of cancer and other diseases, is a story you want to know.

Knowledge of Essiac may change your life. It may give you the knowledge to make more informed decisions for yourself and your loved ones concerning cancer, AIDS, and other prevalent diseases, which threaten every American family. I am hoping that this booklet will also give many of you enough knowledge and interest in the four common herbs of Rene's herbal formula so that you will seek out herbalists who can teach you how to identify, collect and process your own Essiac!

This book is written with the objective of getting

the word out to as many people as possible about
Rene's discovery. Please feel free to copy it and
to give these copies to your friends. If you get as
enthusiastic about Essiac as I am, I am sure that
you will find yourself, as I do, mentioning it to
many of your friends and acquaintances. You
may also, as I do, find yourself taking Rene's
herbal remedy daily as a Preventative and
Detoxifier.

In summary, the information contained herein is
offered to you in the spirit of love and
brotherhood. We hope that you accept it as such,
process the information, and pass it along in the
spirit of love and brotherhood!

In today's society we live with a lot of fear. It
is my hope that your knowledge of Rene's
work may better assist you to live without fear
concerning several of our most dangerous
diseases.

I am not a physician. I am a researcher. I make
no claims that Essiac will cure you. I simply
report to you the information which is already
available in other books and magazine articles.
Make your own conclusions. Consult your
doctor.

Barry

Barry Bryant

Background

Rene Caisse was a nurse in Canada. In 1923 she observed that one of her doctor's patients, a woman with terminal cancer, made a complete recovery. Inquiring into the matter, Rene found that the woman had cured herself with an herbal remedy which was given to her by an Ojibway indian herbalist. Rene visited the medicine man, and he gladly and freely presented her with his tribe's formula. He explained that the Ojibway used their herbal remedy for both spiritual balance and body healing. The formula consisted of four common herbs. They were blended and

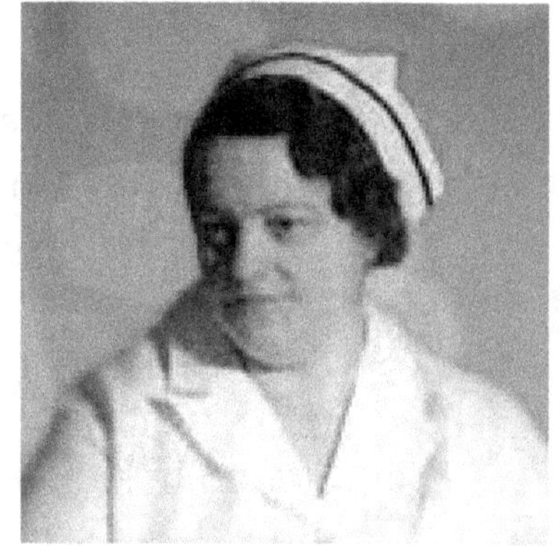

cooked in a fashion which caused the concoction to have greater curative power than any of the four herbs themselves. The four herbs were Sheep Sorrel, Burdock Root, Slippery Elm Bark, and Rhubarb Root.

With her doctor's permission, Rene began to administer the herbal remedy to other terminal cancer patients who had been given up by the medical profession as incurable. Most recovered.

Rene then began to collect the herbs herself, prepare the remedy in her own kitchen, and to treat hundreds of cancer cases. She found that Essiac, as she named the herbal remedy, could not undo the effects of severe damage to the life support organs in some advanced cancer patients. However, the pain of the illness was alleviated and the life of the patients was extended longer than predicted. In the other cases, where the life support organs had not been severely damaged, cure was complete, and the patients lived another 35 or 40 years. Some are still alive today.

Rene selflessly dedicated herself to helping these patients. She continued to treat hundreds of patients from her home. She did not charge for her services. Donations were her only income. They barely kept her above the poverty line. Over the years word of her work began to spread.

The Canadian medical establishment did not take kindly to this nurse administering this remedy directly to anyone with cancer who requested her help. Thus began many years of harassment and persecution by the Canadian Ministry of Health and Welfare. Word of this struggle was carried throughout Canada by newspapers.

The newspaper coverage of Rene's work began to make her famous throughout Canada. Word was also spread by the families of those healed by Essiac. Eventually, the Royal Cancer Commission of Canada became interested in her work. They undertook to study Essiac.

In 1937 the Royal Cancer Commission conducted hearings about Essiac. Their conclusion was that Essiac was a cure for cancer.

Eventually the Canadian Parliament, prodded by the newspaper coverage and the widespread support generated for Rene by former patients and grateful families, voted in 1938 on legislation to legalize the use of Essiac. Fifty-five thousand signatures were collected on a petition presented to the Parliament. The vote was close, but Essiac failed by three votes to be approved as an officially sanctioned cure for cancer.

The complete story of Rene Caisse's life and struggles is told in a book written by Dr. Gary L. Glum entitled <u>The Calling of An Angel.</u> It tells of the documented recovery of thousands of cancer patients who had been certified in writing by their doctors as incurable. Rene continued her work for 40 years until her death in 1978. Rene had entrusted her formula to several friends, one of whom passed the formula along to Dr. Gary Glum.

Of interest is that, in the 1960s, Rene Caisse

worked with the well-known Brusch Clinic in Massachusetts. Dr. Charles A. Brusch was the personal physician for President John Fitzgerald Kennedy. After 10 years of research about Essiac, Dr. Brusch made the following statement: "Essiac is a cure for cancer, period. All studies done at laboratories in the United States and Canada support this conclusion." A testimonial letter from Dr. Brusch is included in this handbook.

Further details of these interesting situations are explained in Dr. Glum's book. Dr. Glum also distributed, free of charge, the complete formula for Essiac along with instructions on how to brew it. This information is also contained in this handbook. We are very indebted to Dr. Glum for his work.

What Essiac Is

Rene Caisse's herbal formula contains four commonly occurring herbs:

Sheep Sorrel (Rumex acetosella).

The leaves of young Sheep Sorrel plants were popular as a cooking dressing and as an addition to salads in France several hundred years ago. Indians also use Sheep Sorrel leaves as a tasty seasoning for meat dishes. They also baked it into their bread. Thus it is both an herb and a food.

Sheep Sorrel belongs to the buckwheat family. It is considered to be a common weed throughout the U. S. It thrives with little moisture, and is a good indicator of acidic soils.

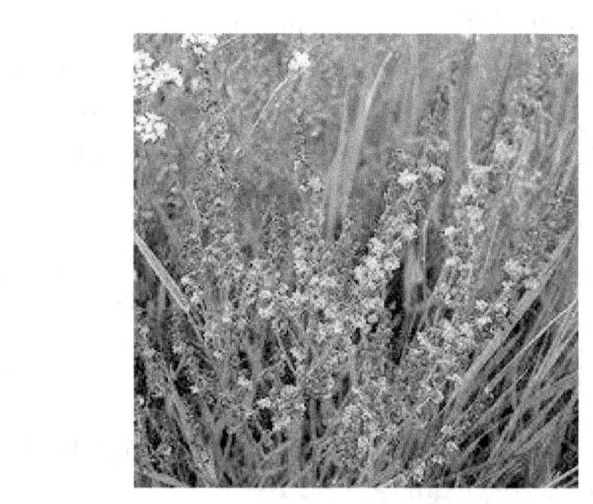

Sheep Sorrel

The entire Sheep Sorrel plant may be harvested to be used in Essiac. Or just the leaves and stems may be harvested, and this allows the plants to be "reharvested" later. The plant portion of the Sheep Sorrel may be harvested throughout the spring, summer, and fall, to be taken early in the morning after the dew has evaporated, or late in the afternoon.

<u>Burdock Root</u> (Arctium lappa).

The roots, young stems, and seeds of the Burdock plant are edible. Young stalks are boiled to be eaten like asparagus. Raw stems and young leaves are eaten in salads. Parts of the Burdock plant are eaten in China, Hawaii, and among the Native American cultures on this continent. It is then, both an herb and a food.

The Burdock is a member of the thistle family. Remember the last time you cleaned cockle burrs from your clothing after a sojourn in the woods or meadow? Chances are, you had run up against this very friendly and helpful plant, you just didn't know it! It is a common pasture weed throughout North America. It prefers damp soils.

The first years the Burdock plant produces only green leafy growth. It is during the second year that it produces the long sturdy stems with annoying burrs.

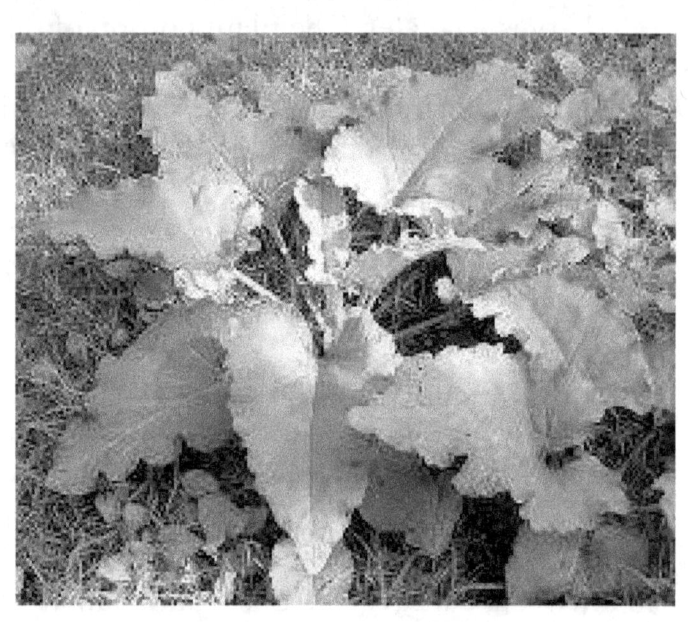

Burdock Root
(It grows up to be the cockleburr plant)

The root of the Burdock plant is harvested. It is harvested from only the first year plants. The roots are about an inch wide, and up to three feet long. As with the Sheep Sorrel, the roots should only be harvested in the fall when the plant energy is concentrated in the roots.

<u>Slippery Elm</u> (Ulcus fulva).

The inner bark of the Slippery Elm tree has a long history of use as a food supplement and herbal remedy. Pioneers knew of it as a survival food. The powdered bark has long been used, and is still being used today, as a food additive and food extender, rich in vitamin and mineral content. Thus it also is a food.

The Slippery Elm is a favorite shade and ornamental tree. It is found throughout Canada and the United States. Only the inner bark of the Slippery Elm is used to make Essiac. Reliable supplies of Slippery Elm can be purchased in powdered form, and this is probably easier and preferable to harvesting it yourself. Should you wish to harvest your own Slippery Elm, strip the bark from branches, rather than from the main trunk system of the tree so that you do not damage the tree.

<u>Rhubarb</u> (Rheum palmatum).

We have all eaten Rhubarb. Its red, bittersweet stems are to be found in supermarket produce shelves each spring. We also eat rhubarb pie, jams and pudding. The roots are used in our tea. The roots are harvested when the plants are at least six years old.

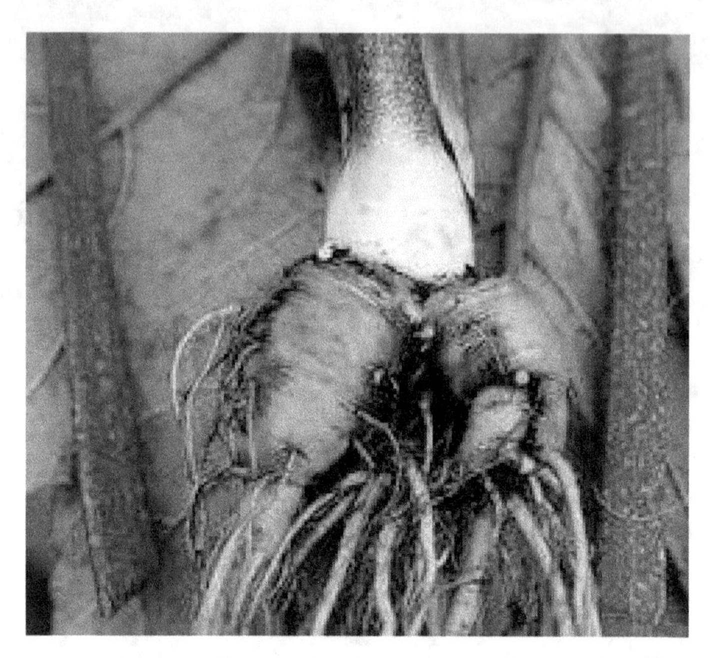

Rhubarb Root

Notes:

1. Should you choose to harvest your own plants, we strongly suggest that you follow the Native American practice of saying a short prayer to the plants before you harvest them. Thank them for the help they will give you. We believe that your plants, thus consecrated, will be more potent and effective.

2. Keep your eye out for classes on herbs and herb identification. Seek out

herbalists who are willing to educate you on plant identity, harvesting techniques, plant drying and processing.

3. Do not collect herbs from areas where insecticides or herbicides have been used. You want only organic herbs!

Additional Herbs

Later in her life, when Rene Caisse worked with Dr. Charles Brusch in Massachussetts, they added four additional herbs in small "potentizing" amounts (this means that they just added these extra herbs in very small amounts). The four extra herbs were:

Red clover
Kelp
Blessed thistle
Watercress

Many of the Essiac products today contain these four extra herbs. I consider this eight herb formula just slightly better than the four herb formula. What is most important is the quality of the herbs that are used, especially the burdock root and the sheep sorrel.

The Formula

Note: Many of you may prefer to purchase a package of the dried herb mixture and brew their own. We provide mail order instructions on page 14. The original formula, as given by Rene Caisse, is listed below. We are reprinting here her exact instructions for a two gallon batch, although you would probably not need such a large amount at one time. A smaller amount is offered in the mail order dried herbal package (see pg. 14) which makes 1/2 gallon of Essiac (which is a two week or four week supply, depending upon whether you take it once or twice daily).

Ingredients:

52 parts: Burdock Root (cut or dried) (parts by weight)

16 parts: Sheep Sorrel (powdered)

1 part: Turkey Rhubarb (powdered) or 2 parts domestic Rhubarb (powdered)

4 parts: Slippery Elm (powdered)

This is the basic four herb formula which was presented to the Royal Cancer Commission in 1937 by Rene Caisse and was found by them to be "a cure for cancer". Later in her life, while working with Dr.Charles Brusch in

Massachusetts, Rene added small potentizing amounts of four other herbs to her basic four herb formula. As provided to us by a woman who worked with Rene, and was given the formula by Rene, these extra four herbs were added as follows: Kelp (2 parts), Red Clover (1 part), Blessed Thistle (1 part), Watercress (0.4 parts). We consider the addition of these four extra herbs optional.

Supplies Needed:

4 gallon stainless steel pot with lid 3 gallon stainless steel pot with lid Stainless steel fine mesh double strainer, funnel & spatula 12 or more 16 oz. sterilized amber glass bottles with airtight caps, or suitable substitutes.

Preparation:

1. Mix dry ingredients thoroughly. Place herbs in a plastic bag and shake vigorously. Herbs

Stir in are light sensitive; keep stored in a cool dark place.

2. Bring 2 gallons of sodium free distilled water to a rolling boil in the 4 gallon pot (with lid on). Should take approximately 30 minutes at sea level.

3. 1   cup

of dry
ingredien
ts.
Replace
lid and
continue
to boil
for 10
minutes.

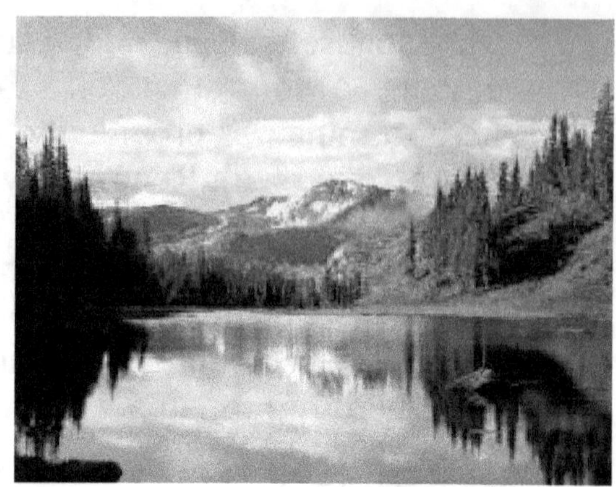

4. Turn off
stove. Scrape
down the
sides of the
pot with the
spatula and
stir mixture
thoroughly.
Replace the
lid.

5. Allow the pot to remain closed for 12 hours.
Then turn the stove to the highest setting and heat
to a boil (approximately 20 minutes). Do not let
boil.

6. Turn off the stove. Strain the liquid into the 3
gallon pot. Clean the 4 gallon pot and strainer.
Then strain the filtered liquid back into the 4
gallon pot.

7. Use the funnel to pour the hot liquid into sterilized bottles immediately, and tighten the caps. After the bottles have cooled, retighten the caps.

8. Refrigerate. Rene's herbal drink contains no preservative agents. If mold should develop, discard the bottle immediately.

Caution: All bottles and caps must be sterilized after use if you plan to reuse them for Essiac. Bottle caps must be washed and rinsed thoroughly, and may be cleaned with a 3% solution of <u>food grade</u> hydrogen peroxide (may be purchased in health food stores). To make a 3% solution, mix 1 ounce of 35% food grade hydrogen peroxide with 11 ounces of sodium free distilled water. Let soak for 5 minutes, rinse and dry. If food grade hydrogen peroxide is not available, use one half teaspoon of Clorox to one gallon of distilled water.

Instructions for Use (as reported by Dr. Glum)

1. Keep refrigerated.

2. Shake bottle well before using.

3. May be taken either cold from the bottle, or warmed (never microwave).

4. As a Preventative, daily take 4 tablespoons (2 ounces) at bedtime or on an empty stomach at least 2 hours after eating.

5. Cancer and AIDS sufferers, or other ill people, may wish to twice daily take 4 tablespoons (2 ounces), once in the morning, 5 minutes before eating, and once in the evening, at least 2 hours after eating.

Note:

    a. Stomach Cancer patients must dilute the herbal drink with an equal amount of sodium free distilled water.

    b. Many people have reported that Rene's drink works well to detoxify the body, and have taken it as a detoxification program.

<u>Precaution</u>: Some doctors advise against taking the herbal formula while pregnant.

<u>Recommendation</u>: Rene reported that the twelve hour brewing process is essential for Essiac to have its special powers. Essiac is being offered to the public in pills, teabags, and homeopathic drops. We do not recommend them. They may work, but they are not what Rene Caisse used, nor have we seen evidence that they work.

What It Does

The components of Rene's herbal drink interact to have an amazing effect on the human body. The chemicals, minerals, and vitamins all act synergistically together to produce a variety of healing agents.

Sheep Sorrel:

Sorrel plants have been a folk remedy for cancer for centuries both in Europe and America. Sheep Sorrel has been observed by researchers to break down tumors, and to alleviate some chronic conditions and degenerative diseases.

It contains high amounts of vitamins A and B complex, C, D, E, K, P and vitamin U. It is also rich in minerals, including calcium, chlorine, iron, magnesium, silicon, sodium, sulfur, and has trace amounts of copper, iodine, manganese and zinc. The combination of these vitamins and minerals nourishes all of the glands of the body. Sheep Sorrel also contains carotenoids and chlorophyll, citric, malic, oxalic, tannic and tartaric acids.

The chlorophyll carries oxygen throughout the bloodstream. Cancer cells do not live in the presence of oxygen. This is important to know. It also:

- reduces the damage of radiation burns
- increases resistance to X-rays
- improves the vascular system, heart function intestines, and lungs
- aids in the removal of foreign deposits from the walls of the blood vessels
- purifies the liver, stimulates the growth of new tissue
- reduces inflammation of the pancreas, stimulates the growth of new tissue
- raises the oxygen level of the tissue cells

Sheep Sorrel is the primary healing herb in Essiac.

Burdock Root

For centuries Burdock has been used throughout the world to cure illness and disease. The root of the Burdock is a powerful blood purifier. It clears congestion in respiratory, lymphatic, urinary and circulatory systems. It promotes the flow of bile, and eliminates excess fluid in the body. It stimulates the elimination of toxic wastes, relieves liver malfunctions, and improves digestion. The Chinese use Burdock Root as an aphrodisiac, tonic, and rejuvenator. It assists in removing infection from the urinary tract, the liver, and the gall bladder. It expels toxins through the skin and urine. It is good against arthritis, rheumatism, and sciatica.

Burdock Root contains vitamins A, B complex, C, E, and P. It contains high amounts of chromium, cobalt, iron, magnesium, phosphorus, potassium, silicon, and zinc, and lesser amounts of calcium, copper, manganese, and selenium.

Much of the Burdock Roots curative power is attributed to its principal ingredient of Unulin, which helps to strengthen vital organs, especially the liver, pancreas, and spleen.

Slippery Elm Inner Bark

Slippery Elm Bark is widely known throughout the world as a herbal remedy. As a tonic it is known for its ability to sooth and strengthen the organs, tissues, and mucous membranes, especially the lungs and stomach. It promotes fast healing of cuts, burns, ulcers and wounds. It revitalizes the entire body.

It contains, as its primary ingredient, a mucilage, as well as quantities of garlic acid, phenols, starches, sugars, the vitamins A, B complex, C, K, and P. It contains large amounts of calcium, magnesium, and sodium, as well as lesser amounts of chromium and selenium, and trace amounts of iron, phosphorous, silicon and zinc.

Slippery Elm Bark is known among herbalists for its ability to cleanse, heal, and strengthen the body.

<u>Rhubarb</u>

Rhubarb, also a well known herb, as been used worldwide since 220 BC as a medicine.

The Rhubarb root exerts a gentle laxative action by stimulating the secretion of bile into the intestines. It also stimulates the gall duct to expel toxic waste matter, thus purging the body of waste bile and food. As a result, the liver is cleansed, and chronic liver problems are relieved.

Rhubarb root contains vitamin A, many of the B complex, C, and P. Its high mineral content includes calcium, chlorine, copper, iodine, iron, magnesium, manganese, phosphorous, potassium, silicon, sodium, sulfur, and zinc.

Rene Caisse's Herbal Drink Has The Following Therapeutic Activity:

1. Prevents the buildup of excess fatty deposits in artery walls, heart, kidney and liver.

2. Regulates cholesterol levels by transforming sugar and fat into energy.

3. Destroys parasites in the digestive system and throughout the body.

4. Counteracts the effects of aluminum, lead and mercury poisoning.

5. Strengthens and tightens muscles, organs and tissues.

6. Makes bones, joints, ligaments, lungs, and membranes strong and flexible, less vulnerable to stress or stress injuries.

7. Nourishes and stimulates the brain and nervous system.

8. Promotes the absorption of fluids in the tissues.

9. Removes toxic accumulations in the fat, lymph, bone marrow, bladder, and alimentary canals.

10. Neutralizes acids, absorbs toxins in the bowel, and eliminates both.

11. Clears the respiratory channels by dissolving and expelling mucus.

12. Relieves the liver of its burden of detoxification by converting fatty toxins into water-soluble substances that can then be easily eliminated through the kidneys.

13. Assists the liver to produce lecithin, which forms part of the myelin sheath, a fatty material that encloses nerve fibers.

14. Reduces, perhaps eliminates, heavy metal deposits in tissues (especially those surrounding the joints) to reduce inflammation and stiffness.

15. Improves the functions of the pancreas and spleen by increasing the effectiveness of insulin.

16. Purifies the blood.

17. Increases red cell production, and keeps them from rupturing.

18. Increases the body's ability to utilize oxygen by raising the oxygen level in the tissue cells.

19. Maintains the balance between potassium and sodium within the body so that the fluid inside

and outside each cell is regulated: in this way, cells are nourished with nutrients and are also cleansed.

20. Converts calcium and potassium oxalates into a harmless form by making them solvent in the urine. Regulates the amount of oxalic acid delivered to the kidneys, thus reducing the risk of stone formation in the gall bladder, kidneys, or urinary tract.

21. Protects against toxins entering the brain.

22. Protects the body against radiation and X-rays.

23. Relieves pain, increases the appetite, and provides more energy along with a sense of well being.

24. Speeds up wound healing by regenerating the damaged area.

25. Increases the production of antibodies like lymphocytes and T-cells in the thymus gland, which is the defender of our immune system.

26. Inhibits and possibly destroys benign growths and tumors.

27. Protects the cells against free radicals.

Essiac and Chronic Fatigue, Lupus, Alzheimer's, Etc.

We have found Essiac to be very helpful to many people with Chronic Fatigue Syndrome, Lupus, Multiple Sclerosis, and Alzheimer's. To the best of our knowledge, all Lupus suffers who have taken Essiac have been significantly helped. We have also witnessed very rapid recoveries among chronic fatigue sufferers. Usually they report a very dramatic increase in energy. Some multiple sclerosis sufferers had less dramatic, but steady improvements in their conditions. One lady put her crutches away after taking Essiac for three months. Alzheimer's sufferers have reported improvements. Some with arthritis have reported improvement, although apparently not all arthritic sufferers are helped by Essiac.

It appears that Essiac's actions to remove heavy metals, detoxify the body, restore energy levels, and rebuild the immune system, all act to restore the body to a level to where it is able to better defeat the illness. In other words, Essiac rebuilds the immune system and improves the illness defeating ability of the body so that it can then rid itself of the illness.

<u>Essiac and AIDS</u>

In 1993 Dr. Gary Glum worked with an AIDS project in Los Angeles. The project had sent 179 AIDS patients home to die. They had pneumocystis carinii and histoplasmosis. Their weight was down and their cell counts were less than ten.

The project gave Dr. Glum five of these patients to work with. He took them off AZT and put them on a protocol of taking 2 ounces of Essiac three times a day. By February of 1994, all of the other patients had died. Dr. Glum's five patients were still alive. They were exercising, eating three meals a day, their weights were back to normal, and they had no appearance of illness.

<u>An Important Endorsement by Dr. Julian Whitaker, M.D.</u>

Dr. Julian Whitaker publishes a very informative and enlightening monthly newsletter named <u>Health & Healing</u>. It has 430,000 subscribers. In his November, 1995 issue he has an article titled "What I Would Do If I Had Cancer". He states that if he had cancer, he personally would follow a regimen which included changing his diet, taking the nutritional supplements Vitamin C, Shark Cartilage, Coenzyme Q1O, and <u>he would take Essiac tea.</u>

Dr. Whitaker has over twenty years of experience. He has written five major health books:

Reversing Heart Disease, Reversing Diabetes, Reversing Health Risks, A Guide to Natural Healing, and Is Heart Surgery Necessary? Dr. Whitaker directs the Whitaker Wellness Institute in Newport Beach, California, which has treated thousands of patients. Should you desire information about subscribing to his newsletter, call (800)705-5559.

I highly recommend this newsletter to anyone who has a serious illness and wishes to become more knowledgeable about the complete range of healing modalities which are available. He also proscribes a 7 step 30 day wellness program "that will turn your life around".

<u>Random Quotes From Rene Caisse:</u>

"Though I worked each day from 9am to 9pm, my work was so absorbing there was no sense of fatigue. My waiting room was a place of happiness where people exchanged their experiences and shared their hope. After a few treatments, patients seemed to throw off their depression, fear, and distress. Their outlook became optimistic and as their pain decreased, they became happy and talkative."

"I could see the changes in some of the patients. A number of them, presented to me by their doctors after everything known to medical science had been tried and failed, being literally carried into my clinic for their first treatment. To later see these same people walk in on their own, after only five or six treatments, more than repaid me for all of my endeavors. I have helped thousands of such people. Some weeks I would have five or six hundred patients. I offered the treatment at no charge."

"Most importantly, and this was verified in animal tests conducted at the Brusch Medical Center and other laboratories, it was discovered that one of the most dramatic effects of taking this remedy was its affinity for drawing all of the cancer cells, which had spread, back to the original site at which point the tumor would first harden, then later soften until it vanished altogether. In other cases, the tumor would decrease in size to where it could be surgically removed with minimal complications. "

Disclaimer:

We have gathered together in this easy-to-read handbook all of the already published information that is available to the general public about Rene's herbal remedy so that you may better make informed decisions. The documents which were used to compile this handbook are listed in the bibliography. Consult your physician before using Rene Caisse's herbal remedy. Copyright 1993 by James Percival. Publishing rights assigned to Bernard Barbieux Associates, Les Tres Peyres, Monbahus, France.

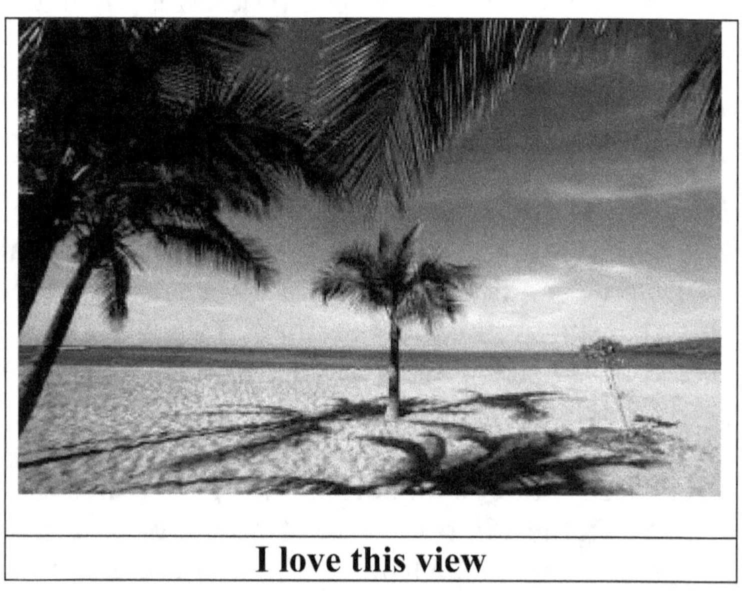

I love this view

Bibliography & Reading List

The Calling of an Angel by Dr. Gary Glum, 1988, Silent Walker Publishing, PO Box 80098, Los Angeles CA, 90080 Tel: (310) 271 9931

The Essence of Essiac by Sheila Snow, 1993

Essiac: Nature's Cure For Cancer: An Interview with Dr. Gary Glum by Elisabeth Robinson, "Wildfire Magazine", Vol. 6, No. 1

Cancer Therapy by Ralph W. Moss, Ph.D., Equinox Press, 331 W. 57th St., Suite 268, New York, NY 10019, 1992

Health & Healing newsletter by Dr. Julian Whitaker, Phillips Publishing, 7811 Montrose Rd., Potomac MD 20854

My Favorite Source to Purchase Essiac Tea:

I purchase my Essiac tea from the following company in the United States. They give me courteous attention when I telephone them, their Essiac tea is made from organic herbs of the highest quality, their service is good, and their prices are fair.

My favorite source for Essiac Tea is **Natural Heritage Enterprises** at
http://www.remedies.net

Crestone CO 81131 USA
Tel: (719) 256 4876 Fax: (719) 256 4874 Toll
Free Telephone: 888-568-3036

—

How To Order: You may place an order on our English language website http://remedies.net . It will be helpful if you have someone who speaks English assist you. You will also have to have a Mastercard, Visa, or American Express credit card. On the website, go to the "Order" button. Then place your order. For faster delivery, we ship to China using postal air service. There will be an extra charge of US$3.00 that will automatically added to your bill to cover the extra air delivery costs to China. This is in addition to the postal charge shown on the website.

Because of the high air mail shipping cost, we do not recommend their liquid Essiac that is in bottles. It is better for you to order the dried herbal packets which are much lighter, and thus more economical to ship to you.

Our Best Ever Testimonial Letter

Charles A. Brusch, M.D.
15 Grozier RD.
Cambridge, Massachusetts 02138

April 6, 1990

TO WHOM IT MAY CONCERN:

Many years have gone by since I first experienced the use of ESSIAC with my patients who were suffering from many varied forms of Cancer.

I personally monitored the use of this old therapy along with Rene Caisse R.N. whose many successes were widely reported. Rene worked with me at my medical clinic in Cambridge, Massachusetts and where, under the supervision of my many medical doctors on staff, she proceeded with a series of treatments on terminal Cancer

patients and laboratory mice and
together we refined and
perfected her formula.
On mice it has been shown to
cause a decided recession of
the mass and a definite
change in cell formation.

Clinically, on patients suffering
from pathologically proven
Cancer, it reduces pain and
causes a recession in the growth.
Patients gained weight and showed
a great improvement in their
general health. Their elimination
improved considerably and their
appetite became whetted.

Remarkably beneficial results
were obtained even an those
cases at the "end of the road"
where it proved to prolong life
and the "quality" of that life.

In some cases, if the tumor
didn't disappear, it could be
surgically removed after ESSIAC
with less risk of mestastases
resulting in new outbreaks.

Hemorrhage has been rapidly
brought under control in many
difficult cases, open lesions of
lip and breast responded to

treatment, and patients with
Cancer of the stomach have
returned to normal activity among
many other remembered cases.
Also,intestinal burns from
radiation were healed and damage
replaced, and it was found to
greatly improve whatever the
condition.

All these patient cases were
diagnosed by reputable physicians
and surgeons.

I do knew that I have witnessed
in my clinic and knew of many
other cases where ESSIAC was the
therapy used, a treatment which
brings about restoration through
destroying the tumor tissue and
improving the mental outlook
which reestablishes physiological
function.

I endorse this therapy even today
for I have in fact cured my own
Cancer, the original site of
which was the lower bowel,
through ESSIAC alone.

My last Pete examination, where
I Aces expedited throughout the
intestinal tract while

hospitalized (August, 1989) for
a hernia problem, no sign of
malignancy was found.

Medical documents validate this.

I have taken ESSIAC every
day since my diagnosis
(1984) and my recent
examination has given me a
clear bill of health.

I remained a partner with Rene
repose until her death in 1978
and was the only person who had
her complete trust and to whom
she confided her knowledge and
"know-howl of what she named
'ESSIAC."

Others have imitated, but a
minor success rate should never
be accented when the true
therapy available.

Executed as a legal document.
/signed/ Charles A. Brusch, MD

**Editor's Note: Dr. Brusch was President
John F. Kennedy's personal physician.**

ESSIAC TESTIMONIALS

In the fall of 1992 my mother who lives in Ohio was told that her throat and lung cancer had reached the point that she only had ninety days left to live. My sister and I began to help her straighten out her affairs. I heard about Mountain Magic Essiac. I sent her some. She drank it for two months. On December 22, she went back to visit the doctor. He thought that she was coming in to say goodby. When he checked her, she was in total remission. I am a nurse, and I kept her x-rays as proof of her recovery.

Ellen Broderick

I started taking your Essiac Tea several months ago. The results have been Profound and Dramatic. Thank you.

My uncle had lung cancer. They gave him six months to live. He started taking Essiac. That was four years ago. He is convinced that the Essiac saved him.

John Randolph

My friend Joe Roberts was in a very bad way with Lupus. He could hardly move about. Some thought he was close to death. I gave him two bottles of Mountain Magic herbal tea (Essiac). He improved, and started taking Essiac. Within a month he looked like a new man, and appeared completely healed.

Martha MylanderGainsville, Florida

I had prostate cancer. My doctor gave me six months. I took Mountain Magic Essiac Tea, as well as several other natural cures. My prostate cancer is gone.

A liquor store manager in Detroit, Michigan

My husband has been through every treatment for his illness, and I am now trying Essiac tea. I thought I would try it first for my various aches and pains, stress, etc. I believe it has done wonders for me so I have started giving him the tea. It won't hurt and maybe his life will be better.

A friend of mine has liver cancer and even though the onco. gave him six months he is now going on two years and says the only thing he takes is Essiac tea. Believe me, he is living proof of its success for him.

Betty at MPIP Bulletin Board

I met a member of the Pioneer Heritage company at a seminar. He told me about Essiac. I had a cancerous condition in my female organs which was causing me a lot of pain. I took the Essiac, my pain went away, and I am now free of cancer. God Bless Pioneer Heritage Enterprises! My eyes are now opened up to the value of natural healing systems, and I spend a lot of time preaching this new religion to my friends.

Marlene Johnson

I am 71 years old. I have had a very rare illness for twenty years. The medical people don't know what causes it, and they don't have a cure. It is called Cogan's Syndrome. It has destroyed my hearing in both ears, caused a lot of vertigo, a lot of aches and pain, and has damaged my heart. Most of my life I have had several colds every year and usually a case of the flu. In January of 1996, the flu turned into pneumonia. That was when I decided to give your Mountain Magic Essiac Tea a try.

I am happy to tell you that since I began using your Mountain Magic I have not had a cold or a sign of the flu. I do believe that it has helped in my recovery from the pneumonia. I plan to continue its use. I drink 2 ounces about three times a week.

Chuck
299 Lake Mamie Rd., Deland FL 32724

My brother-in-law gave me a bottle of Mountain Magic herbal tea to try as a preventive measure. I enjoyed the taste. Soon realized a 20 year stomach problem was gone,. and it gives me an all around better feeling. I am 60 years old and I work 7 days a week.

My nephew in Wisconsin learned he had cancer. He is unable to take Chemo because of other health problems. He takes your tea faithfully; one year later all is in remission. Our family also uses your organic sea salt; my wife used to have water retainage. No longer has a problem there. We enjoy your products and keep up the good work!

Robert W. Heath
9539 Stevenson Rd.
Fenwick MI 48834

I had prostate cancer. On August 10, 1994 I was given chemotherapy. I never told the doctor that I was taking Essiac and as a result the PSA rating went below 0 (zero). I took the combination for 15 months and when it held below zero I quit the chemotherapy. I am continuing taking the Essiac.

Bob Mancini

I have multiple sclerosis. My friend Kelly started me on Essiac. After three months I was able to put my crutches away. After a year, I walk with only a slight limp.

Terry

I am in my fifties. It seems as if all my life I

have had the flu at least once each year, and a bad cold for several times each year. It was like you could just automatically block out 1 to 2 months of each year when I would be laid up with the flu or a bad cold. I started taking Mountain Magic Essiac five years ago. Since that time I have not had the flu, and only had a cold once (I think that the cold was part of a detoxification process). I am sure that Essiac did this for me.

Orlando, Florida

My brother was diagnosed one year ago with very, very severe leukemia. His doctors gave him chemotherapy for four weeks. The chemo made him look deathly ill. My sister and I were appalled. He looked like death itself. This large man, who was over 6 feet tall, lay in his hospital bed in a fetal position, shaking from the chemotherapy.

The doctors told him that he would die in the hospital if he stayed, or he could go home and die. My sister is a nurse, and she was determined to save my brother. She knew of the herbal remedy for cancer called Essiac. She asked the doctor to approve bringing Essiac into the hospital to give to our brother. The doctor felt that there was nothing else he could do, so he paved the way with the medical authorities.

My brother began taking Essiac and 10 drops of Paul 'D Arco herbal formula each day, once in the morning, and once in the evening. His blood count was at 4,800 (10,000 is normal). Within one week of the Essiac treatment he was not only alive, his blood count was at 10,800. In one more week, his blood count was up to 14,000--4,000 higher than normal.

My brother began his Essiac treatments in August, 1992. He was so healthy by the next January that he and his wife went on a four month cruise around the world. It is now August 1993, and he is very healthy, active and robust. I have to withhold my name because I do not want a lot of people calling me about his experience. I love my brother very much, we are very close, and I just thank God for simple things like
Essiac, and the people all over who prayed for his recovery.

Name Witheld

I have a friend from West Virginia who has had rheumatoid arthritis for over 9 years. In May I gave her some of my Essiac. She liked it and began taking it regularly. Within 2 weeks she felt great relief from her pain. Within 2 months she could raise her arms full length over her head, something she had not been able to do for 9 years. She just went to Ireland to visit her relatives, and she took some Essiac with her to give to them.

Bob
Winter Springs FL

Several years ago, I escorted my mother to the outpatient clinic of a local hospital to have a small lump removed from her parotid gland on the left side of her face. What a shock when the doctors found advanced lymphoma cancer throughout her body. I began researching volumes of books looking for some unknown answer. A program of nutritional supplementation and natural food diet was begun, in addition to chiropractic care, positive thought, and humor therapy.

It was extremely tense as the doctors began chemotherapy. In fact, mother was taken to the emergency room six times the first month.

Being 80, it was probably her strong heart that kept her alive and with me to tell her story today. Dancing and teaching others to stay well through dance has kept her going strong all her life.

Letters with prayers for her improved health poured in and a friend sent an article about "Essiac" tea. Hopeful that this herbal formula could somehow help, I went searching for the ingredients, brewed the tea, and added it to her growing list of nutritional supplements.

On Christmas Eve, 1992, three months after my mother's diagnosis of lymphoma, the doctors pronounced that my mother was not just in remission but cancer-free! While we will probably never know what cured her of this dreaded disease, we feel in our hearts that Essiac and nutrition played a major role.

J. Candy Arnold
Bellevue WA

Our family was devastated when my mother-in-law, Myrna, informed us that she had been diagnosed with cancer. In her case, it was ovarian cancer that had spread to the lymph glands and then into the lungs. It was diagnosed as inoperative, and the doctors told her to get her affairs in order. After a hysterectomy, they said, she would have about six months to live. The tumors in her lungs were too numerous to remove. My sister-in-law asked if there was some nutritional approach that might slow the progress of the disease. The doctor assured her there was none. But I nevertheless began to search for alternative remedies. By chance, my father heard a radio program where Essiac was explained.

The remedy was so simple and straightforward that I knew my mother-in-law could take it. She took a little each night. We held our breaths. The doctor and our nurse cousin told us not to get our hopes up. Yet, the weekly x-rays began indicating something they did not expect. Little by little the tumors in her lungs stabilized...and they began to diminish. The nursing staff at the doctor's office reacted in awe as week after week the tumors began disappearing, and her blood count returned to normal.

A little more than a year after beginning Essiac, the doctor called to tell Myrna that she was an official miracle. Her charts showed no indication of cancer in any system. To date, five years later, there has been no recurrence of cancer.

In 2019 my wife Denise was diagnosed with stage 4 breast cancer. She was devastated. I immediately started her on Natural Heritage Enterprises's Essiac tea. She wasn't a big believer in natural cures, but she followed my guidance. We saw progress within a week. She was amazed. Within three months, her tumors had almost vanished. Her doctor was amazed, but he encouraged her to keep up her Essiac regimen. I appreciated this, as many doctors discourage natural remedies.

Well, within six months her doctor pronounced her cancer-free. So now I am a hero to two people; Denise and her doctor! And she religiously takes her Essiac daily as a preventative.

Mike Millard
Colorado

Hi Frank,

That sounds great. How about a box of 24 or whatever fits a shipping box very well? I want to have these available to give to those who do not know about Essiac. Word needs to get out so lives can be saved.

A ladyfriend of ours took Essiac a couple of years ago after I told her about it. She was scheduled for inner ear tumor removal surgery to occur 10 weeks later.

 When she arrived at hospital for surgery the surgeon informed her there would be no surgery because the tumor had vanished.

 Essiac tea and her church friends' earnest prayers saved her health.

 I want more folks to know they can be healed by taking this tea.

If you'll put a box of handbooks together and send an invoice to me, I will happily prepay by PayPal or Visa for the lot plus shipping. Many thanks and best wishes to you.

Carol Hook

PO Box 99

Stanardsville, VA

In 1923 a Canadian Nurse, Rene Caisse, discovered an ancient Ojibway Indian herbal drink that appeared to have remarkable powers to offer the sick.

In the years since, thousands of patients, many considered beyond hope, have testified that this simple natural treatment saved their lives where modern medicine had failed.

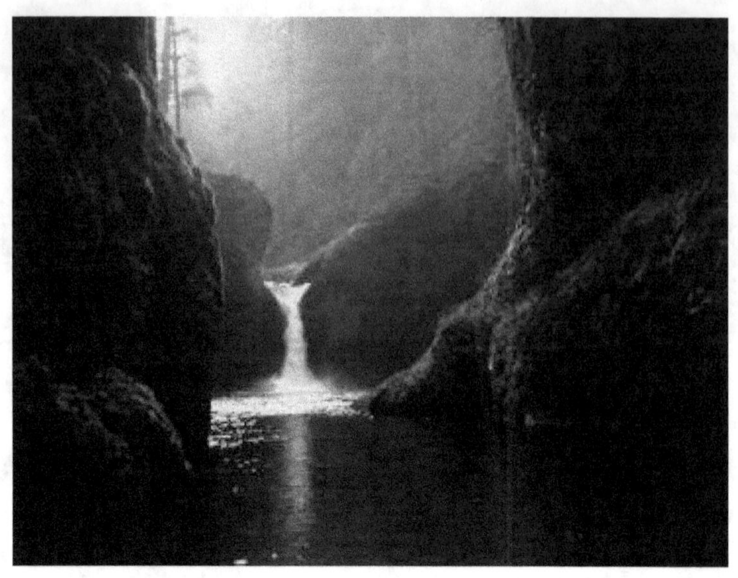

Addendum

1. Using "Structured Water". One of the reasons that we recommend the company Natural Heritage Enterprises (remedies.net) is that they use structured water to make their tea. Here is a short explanation of what structured water is:

Explanation of our Structured Water

We prepare our structured water using principles developed by Dr. Masaru Emoto, Viktor Shauberger and Ed Sopcak, who were all pioneers in this field. The best background information is found in the book *The Hidden Messages in Water* by Dr. Masaru Emoto (and it was a New York Times bestseller for many years).

Our process can be simply described as follows:

1. Dr. Emoto proved that water carries memory. Some of this memory is of a positive vibration, and some of it is of a negative vibration. Our body is 90 percent water.

2. We pass our water thru a device that removes all memory from the water. This method was developed by the owner of the company after studying the work of Dr. Masaru Emoto, and doing 15 years of further research.

3. This water is then passed thru three stations that impart the energies of love and

harmony and gratitude to the water. At this point, the water is all positive energy. We call it "structured water".

4. It is known that negatives attract. When the structured water enters your body (at an all positive charge), it is drawn to the most negative part of your body (where the illness is located). The positive water interrupts the negative energies of the disease , allowing your body's natural healing process to take place.

This is a very simple explanation for a very special and detailed process that changes the nature of the water, making it, as explained in Dr. Emoto's books, into a healing agent.

Additional references:

"Living Energies: An Exposition of Concepts Related to the Theories of Viktor Schauberger" by Callum Coats Jul 19, 2001

"Living Water: Viktor Schauberger and the Secrets of Natural Energy" by Olof Alexandersson   Mar 21, 2002

"The Healing Power of Water" by Masaru Emoto   Sep 1, 2008

On Giving Essiac Tea to your Pets

ESSIAC The Herbal Remedy For Dogs, Cats, Other Pets

Essiac Tea Cures Cancer, Tumors In Dogs, Cats, All Animals

ESSIAC INFORMATION -- Find out all about this fascinating natural cancer remedy and cure for your dog, cat or other pet!

Widely known as an effective alternative medicine remedy for cancer, tumors, and other immune system related illnesses in people, Essiac has also been found effective as a herbal remedy for pets, dogs, cats, other animals. Essiac is inexpensive, easy to take, and Essiac is reported to improve energy levels, as well as build the immune system. If your dog or cat or other pet is suffering from cancer, tumors, feline leukemia, or other immune system illness, or if you are just inquiring about cures for cancer, tumors, or feline leukemia, please check out Essiac tea at our webpage to find out what can be done about the cancer, tumor or other illness your loved pet may be enduring. We encourage you check out Essiac tea and find out about this natural herbal cancer cure and remedy which is available to you.

For some 60 years Essiac has been known to be an effective natural herbal remedy and therapy for cancer in people. We originally began to manufacture and market Essiac to people with cancer. Then we gradually began to discover that Essiac helps a wide range of illnesses in not only people, but pets as well. Dogs and cats, as well as other animals, respond to Essiac. So now we find that immune system illnesses in dogs, cats, and other pets are successfully treated with Essiac. How do we know? Our customers tell us! They report that their dogs and cats recover from cancer, tumors, lupus, infections, leukemia. etc.

We have a number of customers who take Essiac along with their pets.

How do you administer Essiac to your cat or dog or other pet? We suggest that you mix the Essiac tea with an equal amount of water, and place it in your pet's water bowl. They will drink it when they are thirsty. However many of our customers report that they use a syringe to administer the Essiac directly in the animal's mouth.

Substance abuse and Herbal Detoxification

Essiac tea is famous for its detoxifying effects. By detoxifying the body, and especially the liver, our natural herbal tonic has won fame. But its use as a detoxing agent for drug and alcohol substance abuse is also important.

As a herbal cleanser detoxifying drink, the Essiac tea drink provides a natural and smooth way to remove toxins from the body. It is a natural herbal detox for the liver; it has a historical history of helping the blood and the immune system. In short, for those seeking a natural treatment home remedies for alcohol withdrawal, it is a perfect herbal cleanse for detoxifying from alcoholism or drugs.

Those with substance abuse problems often find that cleansing the body of accumulated toxins is essential. Essiac is for you! Our herbal tea drink has a history of assisting the liver to remove accumulated wastes, thus allowing the liver to better do its job of cleansing your body. It is widely recommended among herbal remedies for alcoholic detoxification.

This herbal cleanse is for alcoholics. It is for drug abuse. It is for long-term improvement of the body's immune system defense mechanisms.

Herbal detox for the Liver; the Importance of the Liver and the Defense

Next to the skin, the liver is the largest organ in the body and is often viewed as one of the most critical organs in the human body. As most of you already know, a natural herbal detox cleanse of the liver will assist the alcohol or drug abuse person greatly.

The liver is the organ that stores Vitamin A, D, E and K. The liver metabolizes alcohol The liver is responsible for eliminating and detoxifying the poisons that enter our body The liver produces bile that is essential in the breakdown of fats

In sum, then, it can be seen that alcoholism, sedentary lifestyles, alcohol abuse, environmental pollution, and drug abuse are all factors that lead to the less than optimal functioning of the liver.

Consequences of a Poorly Functioning Liver

The following list represents some of the main outcomes of a poorly functioning liver:

Allergies

Cirrhosis of the liver

Ineffective digestive system

Unhealthy skin

Depressed immune system

Obesity

Alcohol poisoning (due to drinking beyond the ability of the liver to metabolize the alcohol)

Respiratory ailments

Herbal Detox Products and the Liver

There are "natural" ways to augment the overall performance of the liver. One of these ways is the ingestion of herbal detox preparations such as Essiac herbal tea.. This detox, famous for assisting the liver, contains herbs such as sheep sorrel, burdock root, slippery elm bark, rhubarb root, red clover, kelp, blessed thistle and watercress.

It is believed in various "holistic health" groups that herbal detox products rid the liver, colon, and the kidneys of unsafe toxins. It is also believed by these health-advocates that our herbal detox product strengthen the muscles of the large intestine, improve digestion, and assists the gall bladder and the liver.

Building up one's liver via this herbal detox method, therefore, is a slow but sure process that needs to be followed on a daily basis. In short, no herbal detox product will instantly fix your liver; nor will it immediately augment the overall performance of the liver. Given a reasonable amount of time, you will see good results.

For a herbal cleanse detox of your body, how much Essiac tea should you drink? Most of our customers tell us that they take the normal dosage of 2 oz. twice daily on an empty stomach, gradually tapering off to a dosage of once daily.

What About Essiac in Capsule or Pill Form?

A number of years ago, people started putting the dried Essiac herbal mix into capsules or pills and selling these capsules and pills as an easier and more convenient way to take Essiac tea.

The dried herbs that are placed in the capsules have not been brewed.

I do not believe that this is a correct way to take Essiac tea. It must be brewed, and the twelve hour brewing process is critical to the entire process. I have read everything that has ever been written about Rene Caisse and her adventures in developing her Essiac tea.

In her personal writings, Rene Caisse said, "The magic is in the brewing". Enough said. But she added, "When you observe the tea as it goes through the twelve hour setting period after it has been boiled for ten minutes, you will observe that the mixture slowly changes color. I believe that this color change is critical to the effectiveness of the tea."

So I adhere religiously to the original process developed by Rene Caisse. I only use tea that has been brewed and processed according to her original instructions.

What about Essiac for Arthritis and Diabetes?

I get asked these questions often. Yes Essiac tea will benefit people with arthritis and diabetes. However, in all honesty, there is a better way to deal with arthritis and diabetes. It involves dealing with overacidity in the body (which most of us have) and balancing our body's pH down to a healthy level.

There are two small, easy to read booklets that tell you how to deal with these problems. Both are available on amazon.com. One book is **The Diabetes Handbook** and the other book is **Beating Arthritis**. You will be very happy after you have read these books.

How about Lyme Disease?

Wow! Lyme Disease is a nasty business. A friend of mine almost died of it before the doctors finally figured out what his problem was. Hard to diagnose, hard to treat, there are 100,000 people each year who are told that they have Lyme Disease and it is untreatable.

The doctors are wrong. It is treatable. There are herbal formulas that will conquer it. That is how my friend got well.

Again, there is an inexpensive book on amazon.com that explains better than I can, how it works, and how to heal yourself. This is how my friend healed himself. The book is ***The Lyme Disease Handbook***. It is available on amazon.com. It gives the specific herbal formula to use.

Yes, Essiac Tea will help people with Lyme Disease, The rhubarb in the Essiac tea kills parasites, and a bacteria acquired from a tick bite causes the disease. But, frankly, this other herbal formula probably works better.

Here is some additional information that may be of interest to you:

Alternative Medicine Cancer Therapies

That Have Worked For Thousands

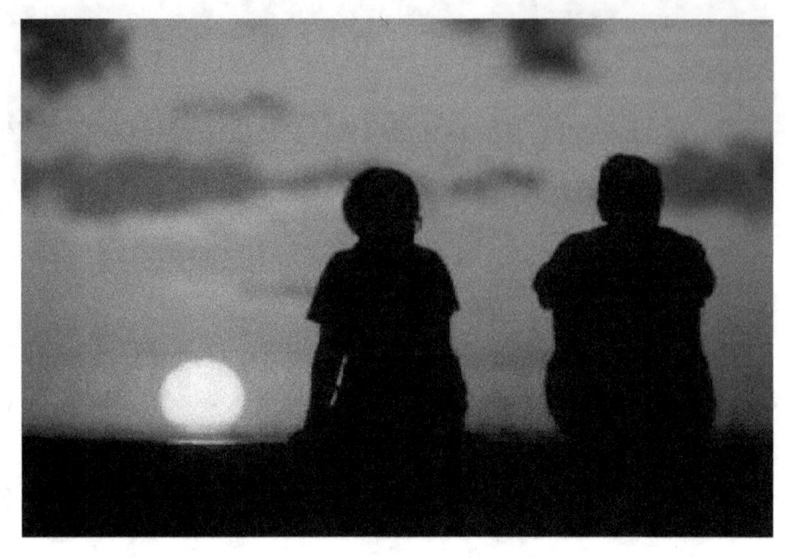

Six Other Natural Cancer Remedies That Are Effective, Inexpensive, And Readily Available

Alternative Medicine Cancer Therapies That Have Worked For Many

Table of Contents

Why You Should Read This Book

The typical practicing physician gets office visits from two categories of people. He gets visited by his patients, and typically he has a waiting room full of patients. He also gets visited, and frequently, by pharmaceutical reps. The pharmaceutical reps are there for several purposes. First, they are there as a reminder for the physician to keep using their company's drug products. But they are there also to brief the physician on their company's latest product developments. They will present the latest technical reports, and sales literature, and free samples, to the doctor. In this way each doctor keeps abreast of the latest developments in his field.

We all know how busy doctors are. The drug company's pharmaceutical reps perform a valuable service to the doctor, and the patients, by keeping the doctor fully informed and educated on the latest developments in the drug industry. The doctor does not have to go home at night and take part of his valuable and scarce private time to study about pharmaceutical advances; he is taught right in his office.

So when you come in to your doctor's office to report that you have cancer, the doctor is already up-to-date on the latest techniques advocated by the pharmaceutical companies for treating cancer. Is it any wonder then that this harried and overworked professional will prescribe a therapy to treat your cancer that follows the recommendations of the pharmaceutical companies? In addition, in medical school he was only taught cancer therapies that were approved by the American Medical Association that is heavily influenced and controlled by the pharmaceutical drug companies. Then, with his busy schedule, he just does not have the time or inclination to search out any natural and inexpensive cancer treatments that might serve you well.

This, of course, does not apply to all doctors. As awareness of the benefits of certain natural alternative cancer therapies become better known among the general populace, many brave doctors are venturing afield into holistic and natural medicines. But to do so places them at risk of censure and ridicule by their peers, as well as formal censure or loss of license to practice medicine.

The point I am making here is that your doctor, for one reason or another, may not tell you all that you need to know about the therapies which would best cure your cancer. So it may be up to you to seek out other sources of information, such as this book.

Those of you who may wish further information about the travails and misfortunes which may befall any doctor who "swims against the current" of conventional medical wisdom should search the Internet for the facts about Dr. Stanislaw Burzynski of Texas, who discovered a cure for certain types of cancer. He has been kept out of prison only because of the widespread support of many other brave physicians who have gone to bat for him. But his career and finances have been ruined because of persecution by the medical establishment.

There is a historical precedent for this type of situation. It took the medical establishment over fifty years to accept antibiotics! Yes, it is true. Penicillin, the first antibiotic, was discovered in the early 1890s. But the medical profession scoffed at the claims made about penicillin, and its use was ridiculed and scorned. It was not until World War II in the 1940s, when the medical profession was overwhelmed with the wounded and injured of war, that penicillin was tried on a mass scale and given a chance to prove its worth. The problem here is that you and I do not wish to wait fifty years for the medical establishment to approve natural effective remedies for cancer.

We do not have the time.

Chapter 1. Oxygen Therapy

The cancer virus is anaerobic. This means that it can only live in the absence of oxygen. As a matter of fact, exposure to oxygen will kill this virus. The HIV virus is anaerobic. Exposure to oxygen will kill it. As a matter of fact, most disease causing viruses are anaerobic. They can only live where there is a low level of oxygen.

This fact becomes most interesting when it is noted that anaerobic viruses can only live in our body when the oxygen carrying capacity of our blood decreases to 60% of its optimum level. This has been known for some time. In 1931 Dr. Otto Warburg was awarded the Nobel Prize for Medicine for his discovery that he had found the cause of cancer to be a lack of oxygen at the cellular level. In 1953 the National Cancer Institute endorsed Dr. Warburg's findings. Additional observations:

Dr. Albert Wahl: "Disease is due to a deficiency in the oxidation process of the body, leading to an accumulation of toxins. These toxins are ordinarily burned in normal oxidation."

Dr. Harry Goldblatt (<u>Journal of Experimental Medicine</u>): "Lack of oxygen clearly plays a major role in causing cells to become cancerous."

Dr. Steven Levine: "Hypoxia, or the lack of oxygen in the tissues, is the fundamental cause of all degenerative diseases."

Dr. John Muntz: "Starved of oxygen the body will become ill, and if this persists it will die. I doubt that there is any argument about that."

There is clearly a correlation between the levels of oxygen in our body and illness. It is important to note that <u>fear, anxiety, worry, and depression</u> all interfere with the breathing process, and will reduce the oxygen intake. This can lead to illness. But there is an even greater problem facing our bodies and their needs for an adequate supply of oxygen. It concerns the very air we breathe.

<u>The Oxygen Story</u>

Remember the movie Jurassic Park? In this movie, Scientists extracted DNA from the blood of mosquitoes, which were imbedded in fossilized amber in order to recreate prehistoric animals. Well, something similar has happened in real life. In the laboratory, real life scientists have extracted air, which was trapped as bubbles in fossilized amber. When the air was analyzed, it was found to contain 38% oxygen. This is very noteworthy because the air we breathe today has an average oxygen content of 21% or less.

The significance of this is immense. As man has evolved from his primitive prehistoric form, <u>the oxygen levels of the air he breathes have dropped 50%</u>. The implications of this on our health may be staggering. What if the human body was designed to live and prosper on air that contained 38% oxygen, a level that is 50% higher than the air we breathe today? What if the reduced levels of oxygen in the air we breathe today are causing our bodies to not receive an adequate level of oxygen for them to be well and healthy?

In fact, the air in various areas of the world is declining in oxygen content. In other words, this situation is getting worse. In some of the larger, more pollution plagued cities, the oxygen levels of air have declined as low as 15%. Man cannot live at levels at 7% oxygen or lower, even for a short period of time. It is safe to say that mankind may be facing a serious problem here.

Other Problems

We do not plan to go into great detail here about the other conditions in our lives, which result in our blood not carrying an adequate supply of oxygen to the muscles and cells of our bodies. In general, we have depleted our soils by the overuse of chemical fertilizers, resulting in our foodstocks not providing us with adequate nutrition. Example: Vegetables today have only 25% of the minerals and enzymes of vegetables grown 90 years ago. And many of the fruits and vegetables come to us contaminated with insecticides and pesticides. The consumption of processed salt, which has 82 of its 84 minerals and trace elements removed, and is coated with aluminum hydroxide which makes it insoluble in our bodies, harms our health. Most of the meat we consume today contains growth hormones and antibiotics, giving new meaning to the expression "you are what you eat." All of these factors lead to a lower level of overall health and energy, and a condition where our weakened bodies become overloaded with toxins. It is the job of our blood to extract these toxins from the cells of our bodies, and carry the toxins to the wall of the large intestine (colon). There the toxins are passed through the wall of the intestine, to be carried away with the waste products of our body.

But there is a problem here. The long-term consumption of too many processed foods has resulted in our large intestines becoming sluggish, which has led to a buildup on the intestinal walls of a hardened mucous-like coating. The average 50 year-old-American Male has a coating lining his colon, which weighs 5 pounds! It acts like a barrier between the wall of the large intestine (colon) and the waste products passing through the colon. As a result, the blood is not able to easily pass the toxins it is carrying through the wall of the colon. Unable to unload its toxins, the blood is forced to continue carrying the toxins. Under better conditions, the blood, after unloading its load of toxins, would pick up a load of oxygen to carry to the cells on its return trip. But now, still loaded with toxins, the blood is unable to carry oxygen back to the body's cells. Oxygen starvation results.

The Symptoms of Oxygen Deficiency

Doctors and scientists have identified the initial symptoms of oxygen deprivation, which actually constitutes the gradual oxygen starvation of the body's seven trillion cells. In addition to illness, these symptoms are:

- overall body weakness
- muscle aches
- depression
- fatigue
- arthritis

- circulation problems
- poor digestion
- lowered immunity to colds, flu, infection
- bronchial problems
- tumors and deposit buildups

- irrational behavior

- irritability & dizziness
- memory loss
- hostility

- bacterial, viral and parasitic infestations
- circulation problems

- acid stomach

People rarely suspect that the above conditions, or the constant vague feelings of helplessness, fatigue or despair is the result of the cells of their body desperately sending out signals that they need more oxygen.

The Use of Oxygen Therapies

By now I hope that I have convinced you of the need to get more oxygen to the cells of your body. You have probably surmised that if we could add oxygen directly to the blood in your body, most

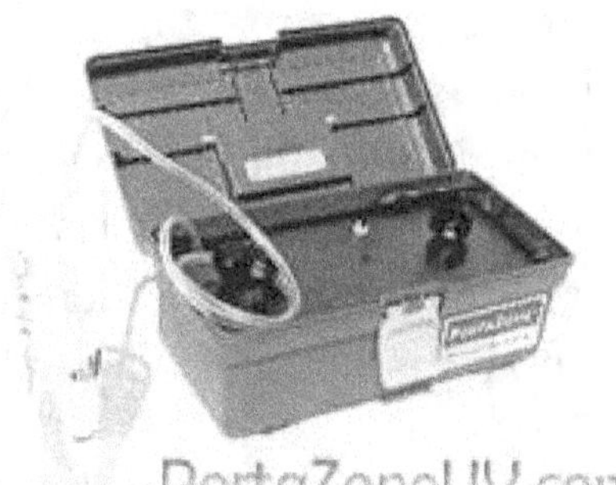

Ozone machines have become portable and affordable

of the disturbing problems discussed above could be overcome. You are right. There are a number of ways to accomplish this. One approach is ozone therapy. Regular oxygen is O2. Ozone is O3, that is, each molecule has an extra atom of oxygen. When ozone is added to your body, the extra oxygen atom immediately leaves the ozone, and attached itself to a cell of your body. Your oxygen level is thereby increased. Chemically, the ozone (O3) has become oxygen (O2) plus oxygen (O). Ozone Therapy is widely practiced in other countries. In Germany, equipment and procedures have become refined to the point that doctors there can remove sluggish, toxin loaded blood from your body, ozonate the blood, remove the toxins, and reinsert the now oxygen enriched blood back into the patient's body. Other less complicated procedures involve using a relatively simple ozone machine to add ozone to the body through rectal insufflations, use of body wraps, or by simply drinking ozonated water. Wondrous cures for a wide litany of illnesses have been effected with ozone therapy. However, ozone therapy is not practiced in the United States.

Another procedure is the use of food grade hydrogen peroxide (H2O2). When hydrogen peroxide is added to the body, the H2O2 quickly becomes H2O (water) plus O (oxygen atom). The oxygen atom attaches itself to a cell of your body, and again, your oxygen level has just gone up. It is <u>very important</u> here to note that the type of hydrogen peroxide (3%), which is typically sold in drug stores and grocery stores, <u>cannot be used</u> for such a purpose. It contains contaminants and is dangerous for such use. Food Grade Hydrogen Peroxide (35%) is available through many health food stores. Food Grade Hydrogen Peroxide is the only type of hydrogen peroxide that can be used. Diluted Food Grade Hydrogen Peroxide can be given intravenously, or absorbed through the skin, or injested. One method which has successfully been used by many is to add 4 to 6 ounces of Food Grade 35% hydrogen peroxide to a tub of hot water and soak for 45 to 60 minutes. This is done daily. The hydrogen peroxide passes thru the skin into the blood stream where it is converted into oxygen. Miraculous recoveries from cancer, arthritis, Epstein Barr, chronic fatigue, lupus, multiple sclerosis, diabetes, allergies, and many other illnesses have been reported.

<u>Why Doesn't Your Doctor Tell You This?</u>

All oxygen therapies, including hydrogen peroxide therapy, are non-patentable processes. They are for the most part also inexpensive, and in many cases can be administered at home by the patient. Therefore there is no financial incentive for the pharmaceutical industry or the American Medical Association to promote these therapies. As a matter of fact, they will discipline severely any doctor caught using oxygen therapy.

This is not the case in certain other countries. In Germany, Russia, and Cuba, for example, physicians have successfully treated many serious and chronic conditions. Cancer, heart disease, AIDS, chronic fatigue, and many other illnesses have been successfully treated. In these countries a treatment consisting of a medical infusion of hydrogen peroxide costs approximately $10. No financial incentive here for the pharmaceutical industry, medical centers, and physicians who are accustomed to providing expensive drugs, and complex medical procedures. Thus, knowledge of this esoteric field is restricted to those intellectually courageous individuals who venture into the realms of alternative medicine.

What Can Be Done?

We have reviewed all of the oxygen therapy methods available, analyzed the cost and practicality of their application, and have reached a conclusion. Drinking water that contains a minute amount of food grade hydrogen peroxide is a good procedure. Many people have significantly increased the oxygen content of their blood, thereby improving their health or overcoming their illness, by this simple protocol. First of all, as we emphasize, use only 35% Food Grade Hydrogen Peroxide. Keep it in the refrigerator, or in a cool dark place (light will damage it). Use only distilled water, or reverse osmosis filtered water. This is because the iron content of regular water will react with the hydrogen peroxide to impart an unpleasant taste to the water. Carefully place 10 drops of the 35% hydrogen peroxide in an 8 oz. glass of distilled water, and immediately drink. Drink 5 glasses of this peroxide water daily. Best if taken on an empty stomach (it will taste better). That's it. Simple and cheap. And effective. Also, soaking daily in a tub of water to which 4 to 6 oz. of food grade hydrogen peroxide has been added, as already mentioned above, is a good therapy.

Mail Order Sources of Food Grade 35% Hydrogen Peroxide

Your local health food store may stock 35% food grade hydrogen peroxide. If not, you may obtain it from:

1. Sullivan Creek Distributing Co., 955 73rd Ave. NE. Carrington ND 58421, Toll Free

Telephone: 888-406-4066, sells a 16 oz. bottle of food grade 35% hydrogen peroxide for $16.95.
2. Raw Health Inc., 11355 SW 14th St, Beaverton OR 97005, Telephone 866-729-4584, sells a 32 oz. bottle of food grade 35% hydrogen peroxide for $18.00.
3. Pure Health Systems, Telephone 970-731-9724 sells 35% food grade hydrogen peroxide. A 16 oz. bottle is $16.95 and a gallon bottle is $55.00.

Note: We are researchers, not physicians. Consult your physician. This researched information does not make any claims. It is not intended to replace sound medical advice.

Additional Reading

For additional reading, Crossroads, Toll Free Tel: 800-635-5823 sells books about oxygen therapy. I recommend *Oxygen Therapies* by Ed McCabe, and *Hydrogen Peroxide and Ozone* by Conrad LeBeau (only $3.95).

<u>**Bibliography**</u>

<u>Oxygen</u> by Dr. Kurt Donsbach, The Rockland
Corporation, Tel: 800 421 7310

<u>Bio/Tech News</u>, newsletter, PO Box 30568,
Parkrose Center, Portland OR 97294

<u>The Story of Ozone</u>, Plasmafire Intl., 7186-205
St. Langley, B.C., V2Y1T1 Canada

<u>Oxygen Therapies</u> by Ed McCabe, $14.00 from
<u>Books</u>, 4100 Bonita Rd. Santa Monica CA 91902

<u>Alternatives</u> newsletter by Dr. David G.Williams,
PO Box 829, Ingram TX 78025

<u>Health & Healing</u> newsletter by Dr. Julian
Whittaker, Phillips Publishing, 7811 Montrose
Rd., Potomac MD 20854

Chapter 2. Kombucha the Amazing Mushroom Tea

Years ago the Russian government sent a team of investigators to check out why the residents of an area in Manchuria were cancer free. The people of this area also regularly lived to be over 100 years of age. After a two-year study, the investigators attributed the longevity and good health of these people to a yeast enzyme tea called Kombucha. It had been part of their diet for hundreds of years. Now the use of Kombucha has been spreading like wildfire in the United States.

In an April, 1995 issue of <u>US Today</u> newspaper, an article about Kombucha tea stated that five to six million Americans were drinking Kombucha tea daily. I am sure that this number of Kombucha drinkers has grown since then. It is inexpensive, I find it fun to make, and most people enjoy the taste. I keep several one gallon "sun tea" jars of Kombucha brewing at all times. I keep the jars prominently sitting on my kitchen counter, where they become a conversation piece for my visitors.

During an August, 1995 TV program of <u>Entertainment Tonight</u> which covered
Kombucha, it was
mentioned that the
Hollywood stars Cher,
Susan Sarandon, Martin
Landau, Meg Ryan and
Linda Evans were all
Kombucha drinkers. In
addition, Anjelica
Huston, Lily Tomlin,
Morgan Fairchild, and
Rita Coolidge are said
to be Kombucha fans. It

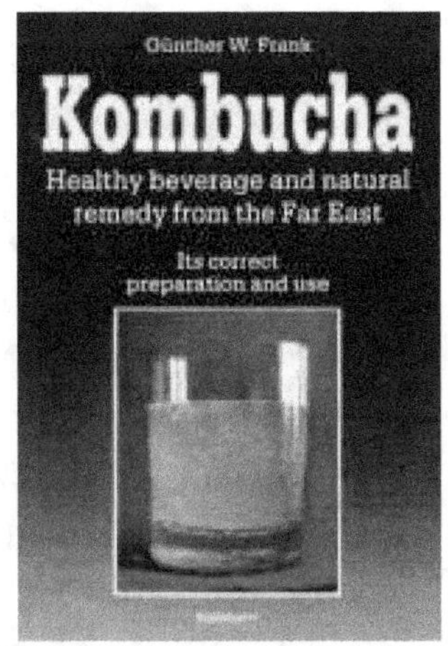

is reported that Kombucha cleanses the blood,
stops cancer, increases energy levels, reverses
hardening of the arteries, reduces high blood
pressure, boosts T-cell counts, removes wrinkles,
thickens the hair, and relieves headaches. Studies
in California report that HIV patients drinking
Kombucha do not progress into AIDS. Other
testimonials state that it reverses graying hair,
stops PMS, reverses the symptoms of multiple
sclerosis, and shrinks prostates.

Kombucha is known to provide the liver with
glucuronic acid, a substance that the liver uses to
detoxify our bodies. In this manner, Kombucha
helps the liver to perform its critical function of
"binding up" toxic substances so they can be

carried away by the blood and dispelled from our bodies.

Amazom.com on the Internet sells a number of books about Kombucha. There is also the book ***"Kombucha: Healthy Beverage and Natural Remedy from the Far East"*** by Guenther Frank which can be purchased from Pronatura, Inc. at 847-545-1003.

Kombucha has been around for centuries without causing any known widespread ill effects. Although newly discovered in the United States, there has been plentiful research done in Europe and Asia confirming its healthful benefits. Kombucha is fun to make, tastes great, is cheap, and if you take it daily, you too may live to become 100 years old.

Sources of a Kombucha Starter Kit

1. Mt. Nebo Herbs & Oils, 300 Highland Ave., Athens OH 45701, Tel: 740-592-3795 sells a Kombucha starter kit, including Kombucha mushroom and full instructions for $15.50 plus $6.95 for Shipping.

2. 2. Laurel Farms, PO Box 2896, Sarasota
    FL 34230, Tel: 941-351-2233 sells a
    Kombucha starter kit, including Kombucha
    mushroom and full instructions, for $39.00
    including Shipping and Handling.

3. Nancy Adams, Ph.D., Tel: 541-888-5111,
    sells a Kombucha starter kit for $15.00
    including Shipping.

Note: These starter kits are all that you will need
to produce a lifetime supply of Kombucha tea.

Chapter 3. Pycnogenol and Grape Seed Extract

An excess of free radicals in a person's body
causes major damage, including cancer. Free
radicals can attack, damage, and ultimately
destroy any material including the sensitive cells
and tissues in the body. The best free radical
killer is Pycnogenol (pronounced pig-nodge-a-
nol). Pycnogenol is a patented antioxidant from
France that is made from a pine tree bark extract.

Let's talk more about free radicals. The normal oxygen atom in your body has four pairs of electrons. However the effects of radiation, sunlight, air pollution, harmful chemicals, food additives, tobacco smoke, infections and stress can rob one of the electrons from the

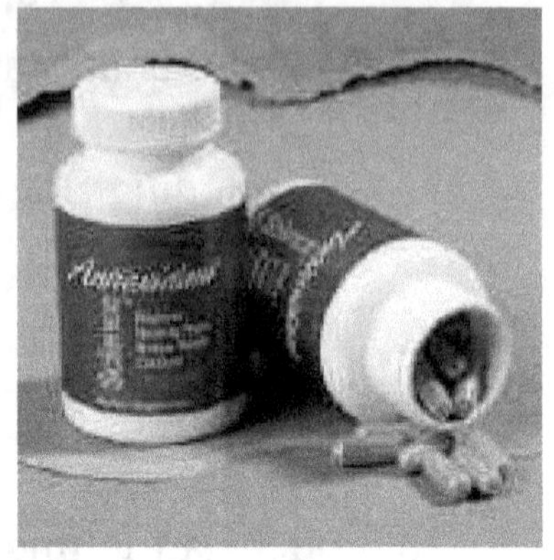

oxygen atom. This atom is now a free radical. It tries to replace its lost electron by raiding other molecules. It will rob an electron from a molecule in a cell wall. This robbed molecule proceeds to replace its lost electron by robbing another molecule, and a chain reaction is created. This leads to disintegration of the cell, and opens the door to cancer and many other ills. It also alters the DNA which damages the way in which the cells in your body replicate. This leads to aging. Some studies suggest that these free radicals are a major cause of aging.

How does Pycnogenol help? It is a very powerful antioxidant. An antioxidant has extra electrons that it can "give up" to the

> Pycnogenol & Grape Seed Extract can be found at your Health Food Store

free radicals, thereby rendering them harmless.

I recommend Pycnogenol because of its power. It has the ability, in a matter of a few months, to destroy all of the excess free radicals that you have built up over a lifetime. It is inexpensive. It is easy to locate. It comes in tablet form. Every health food store stocks it. Dr. Lamar Rosquist recommends that you take one mg. of Pycnogenol daily per pound of body weight during the initial period when you are ridding yourself of all accumulated free radicals. This means that a 200 pound man would take 200 mg. of Pycnogenol daily for the first two or three months. Later you may wish to slack off to a lower maintenance-level dosage.

Pycnogenol is reported to assist in the recovery of cancer, Alzheimers, arthritis, Parkinsons, rheumatism, asthma, diabetes, stress, varicose veins, phlebitis, PMS, AIDS, senility, M.S., chronic fatigue, stroke, circulatory and cardiovascular problems. It adds energy. It has also been reported to greatly assist in limiting wrinkling and aging of the skin.

When I took Pycnogenol, I found my energy levels dramatically boosted.

Grape Seed Extract is reportedly as good as Pycnogenol as a free radical killer. To locate a source of Pycnogenol or Grape Seed Extract, I suggest that you visit one or more health food stores. They may be able to offer some helpful advice, and they may have literature available with additional information about this antioxidant. I have even found Pycnogenol and Grape Seed Extract stocked in K Mart and my local drug store.

Sources of Pycnogenol and Grape Seed Extract

Nature's Rx, 119 Spinnaker Circle, Madison AL 35758, Toll Free Tel: 800-303-5781 sells Grape Seed Extract. A bottle of 90 caplets (90mg per cap) costs $12.00.

Nutri Team, Ripton VT 05766, Toll Free Tel: 800-785-9791 sells Grape Seed Extract. A bottle of 120 caplets (100 mg per cap) costs $11.95.

Primary Source, Inc., PO Box 812, Fairfield CT 06430, Toll Free Tel: 888-666-1188 sells a product named OPC that contains both Pycnogenol and grape seed extract. A bottle of 60 caplets (100 mg per cap) costs $44.95.

Chapter 4. Colon Health and Cancer

Almost everyone remembers that John Wayne died of cancer. When an autopsy was performed on him, it was found that his colon (large intestine) was six inches in diameter and weighed 60 pounds empty. The hole in the center of the colon through which his food passed was one inch in diameter. The large intestine of the average person is about 5 feet long, and is 2.5 inches in diameter. John Wayne's enlarged colon was so packed with an accumulation of undigested and solidified food that there was no way in which he could have lived. I say that John Wayne died of an unhealthy colon, because cancer is only one of the results of an unhealthy and blocked colon.

One of the functions of the blood in your body is
to carry oxygen and nutrients to each cell in your
body. The blood, after delivering this oxygen and
nutrition to each cell, then picks up the waste
product of the cell and carries it to the wall of the
colon. There the waste products are passed
through the wall of the colon, to be carried out of
the body with the next bowel movement.

However, if the
interior walls of
the colon have
become coated
with solidified
food and waste,
this coating on the
wall of the colon
will block the
passage of the
blood's load of
waste products.
Thus, this function
of passing the blood's load of cell waste cannot
be performed. The blood, not able to unload its
load of waste products, will begin to carry it
around the body. Loaded down with this load of
toxic waste products, the blood is not able to pick
up a full load of oxygen and nutrients to resupply
the body's cells. Starved of the necessary oxygen
and nutrients, the body's cells begin to

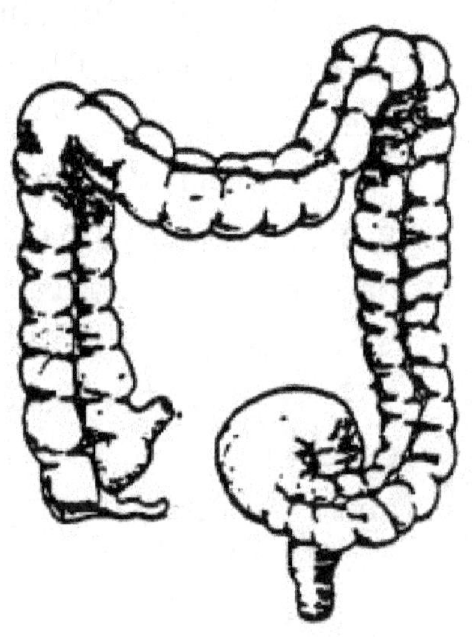

deteriorate. This leads to a host of unhealthy conditions, including eventually cancer. Remember, in Chapter 1 we discussed that cancer can only exist in an environment where there is a lack of oxygen. So it is that the state of health of your large intestine (colon) has a lot to do with whether or not you get cancer.

It is a medical fact that the average American male has a coating of solidified food lining the inside walls of his colon which weighs five pounds! How does this happen? A lifetime of eating too many fatty foods, a diet not containing enough fiber, and too many processed foods in our diet are the culprits. The eventual result of our years of improper eating is that deposits begin to accumulate on the walls of the colon, eventually leading to serious health situations, as emphasized by the example of John Wayne.

Symptoms of an Unhealthy Colon

As we get older, we begin to experience the symptoms of aging. But many times, these are not the symptoms of the normal aging process, they are symptoms of a plugged up colon. We just mistake them as signs of the normal aging process. Symptoms of an unhealthy colon are:

Fatigue	Depression	Anxiety or worry
Gas or Flatulence	Protruding Abdomen	Insomnia
Not feeling good	Lack of interest	Abdominal discomfort
Headaches	Aches and pains	Menstrual problems
Irritability	Loss of memory	Skin problems
Nervousness	Overweight	Bad breath
Nausea	Craving for food	Feel cold (hands and feet)

What Can Be Done?

Obviously, changing your diet to minimize fats and processed foods, and adding fiber, will be required in order to correct the conditions of an unhealthy colon. But if you have cancer, you cannot afford to wait for the months or years it may take to correct the problem. You need to fix your colon now. The answer is Colonics.

What is a Colonic?

A Colonic is much like an enema, except that it is much more thorough and effective. In a 45-minute session, approximately 15 gallons of water is used to gently flush the colon. Through appropriate use of massage, pressure points, etc., the colon therapist is able to work loose and eliminate far more toxic waste than any other short-term technique.

What will Colonics do for the colon ?

Specifically, a Colonic is used to accomplish the following:

1. It cleanses the Colon: Toxic material is broken down so it can no longer harm your body or inhibit assimilation and elimination. Even debris built up over a long period is gently, but surely removed in the process of a series of treatments. Once impacted material is removed, your colon can begin again to co-operate as it was intended to. In this very real sense a colonic is a rejuvenation treatment.

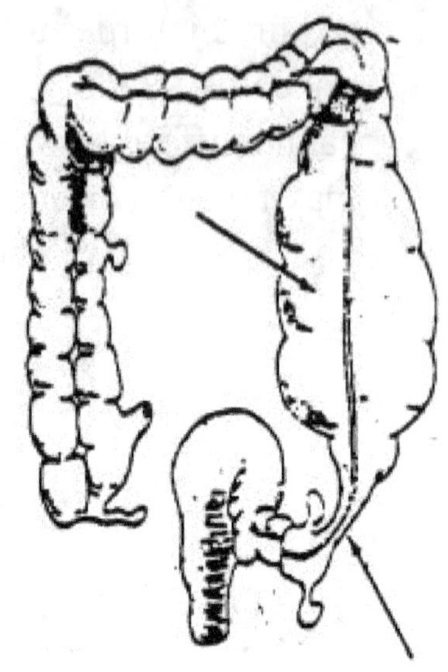

2. It Exercises the Colon Muscles: The build up of toxic debris weakens the colon and impairs it's functioning. The gentle filling and emptying of the colon improves peristaltic (muscular contraction) activity by which the colon naturally moves material.

3. It Reshapes the Colon: When problem conditions exist in the colon, they tend to alter its shape which in turn causes more problems. The gentle action of the water,

An unhealthy colon; note distended and shriveled areas

coupled with the massage techniques of the colon

therapist helps to eliminate bulging pockets of waste and narrowed, spastic constrictions. This enables the colon to resume its natural state.

4. It Stimulates Reflex Points: Every system and organ of the body is connected to the colon by reflex points. A colonic stimulates these points, thereby affecting the corresponding body parts in a beneficial way.

When the lower intestinal tract is cleansed, the whole system is detoxified. Proponents of colon irrigation claim that it actually heals their bodies. Toxicity is a major cause of illness, disease and feelings of general malaise. While colon therapy does not heal any specific disease, it greatly enhances the body's ability to function at optimum levels, so the body is more able to heal itself.

When a system has experienced abusive treatment it has had to endure over a lifetime, toxic waste builds up in the colon and the body cannot properly assimilate the vitamins and minerals we need. The walls of the colon tend to develop a buildup of material and this results in sluggish bowel movements, constipation and other problems. Instead of being expelled correctly, the poisons re-enter the blood stream and circulate through the body. If you are experiencing flatulence, stomach bloat, lower backache, bad breath, stiff joints, mood swings, skin problems, abdominal discomfort, restless sleep, excessive mucous, nausea, constipation, diarrhea, fatigue depression or cloudy urine, you may need to have your colon cleansed. These are signs of an impacted colon.

Many people are under the false impression that an enema is as cleansing as a colonic. An enema only uses 1 to 2 quarts of water while colonic irrigation uses 12 to 15 gallons of water. During the colonic the water travels the whole 5-foot length of the colon, cleaning it from the sigmoid to the ascending colon. The whole colonic treatment is not necessarily limited to the colonic irrigation. Also included usually is abdominal massage and reflexology that is used to stimulate pressure points of the feet that also help with the elimination process. The entire procedure should take 35 to 40 minutes.

The effect of a colonic is not just on the colon. Once your body is detoxified through the colonic irrigation, the other organs of the body work better. It facilitates the cleansing of the blood, liver and the lymphatic system and makes it easier for organs to release their waste products for elimination. Many people claim they suffer from headaches much less after having a colonic treatment. Other benefits that are reported are improvement in appearance, mental attitude, skin tone, and stress is relieved. Constipation and abdominal pain are often eliminated and the old feeling of exhaustion is replaced with a feeling of energy. And if you have cancer, the glands and organs of your body will function better, causing your immune system to work better, and be able to better combat the cancer in your body.

Where Can I Get a Colonic?

Good places to locate a colon therapist who will administer a colonic are your local health food store bulletin board and the telephone book yellow pages. You may also wish to ask about among the health-conscious. One of them will be able to recommend a good colonics specialist to you.

Chapter 5. Cancer and the Parasite Connection

Dr Hulda Clark is a medical researcher from Canada. She is convinced that many diseases, especially cancer, result from the invasion of parasites in the colon.

From this simply stated but well researched idea, she has written a series of books and produced a range of products and recommendations which have resulted in a huge following in the United States of America and in many other countries.

Her first best selling book " The Cure for all Cancers" has been followed by "The Cure for all Diseases", and she has developed her ideas and her following by the good results her patients are experiencing. Dr Clark believes that if the body can be rid of colon parasites it can restore itself to full health. Dr Clark recommends a combination of herbal parasite cleanses, the use of her inexpensive electronic "zapper", and kidney and liver flushes as the best possible ways to rid the body of colon parasites.

How is it that a parasite can cause cancer?

Unknown to most of
us, most people have
one or more types of
parasites in their
bodies. They got
them from running
barefoot as children,
from eating
undercooked meat, from
eating improperly washed

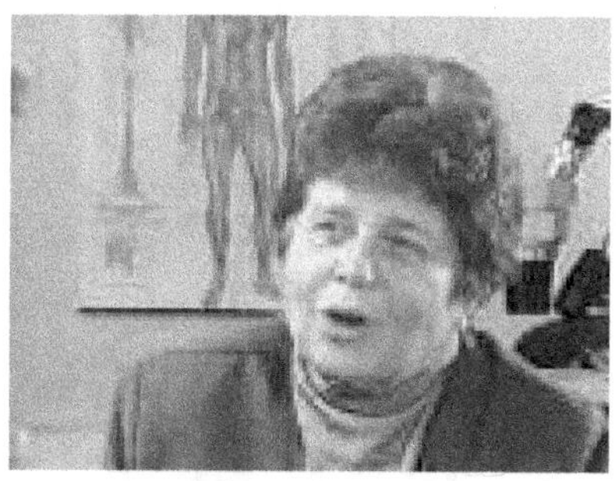

Dr. Hulda Clark

fruits and vegetables, and from handling pets.
One of these parasites is an intestinal fluke. Its
scientific name is *Fasciolopsis buskli*. It is quite
small. Normally this fluke lives in our intestinal
tract, where it does little harm. But sometimes,
over years without detection or treatment, these
flukes multiply to the point where they begin to
travel outside the colon to other parts of the body.
Sometimes they invade other organs or parts of
the body. There they do a great deal of harm.
There they can cause cancer.

For example, let us assume a situation where
these intestinal flukes have invaded and
established themselves in a liver. There they
multiply until there may be thousands of flukes.
These flukes are all busy devouring your body
fluids and nutrients, and in turn spewing out their
waste products. These waste products
contaminate your liver. There is a growth factor
in your liver that is called ortho-phospo-tyrosine.

For brevity I shall refer to it as "ortho". This ortho has a normal function of causing cells to divide. But the fluke's waste products cause the ortho to sometimes go haywire, and the ortho causes cells to divide where they shouldn't. This leads to improperly growing cells, which often leads to cancer.

Why Cancer Locates Where It Does

Why does one person develop cancer in the lungs, and another person develop cancer in the kidneys? It is because this particular area of the body is weakened. Generally, parasites thrive better in a weakened organism. So the flukes will be attracted to this weakened area of the body. Eventually a cancerous condition will develop.

Why is this particular part of the body weakened? Because it probably has a number of the following problems:

a. has low immune power

b. accumulated a heavy dosage of heavy metals

c. accumulated a large dosage of toxins

d. receives improper nutrition

e. does not receive enough oxygen

f. has too many free radicals.

Let's Get Rid Of The Parasites!

Dr. Hulda Clark recommends the following protocols to get rid of the parasites in your body:

1. A Herbal Parasite Cleanse. Dr. Clark recommends a combination of Black Walnut Hull extract, Wormwood and Cloves. My favorite source for these parasite-removing products is the company founded by Hanna Kroeger, a famous herbalist. It is Kroeger Herbal Products, 805 Walnut St., Boulder CO 80302, Toll Free Tel: 800-516-0690. Tell them what you wish to do, and they will advise which products to buy and how to take them. They are very honest people.

2. The "Zapper". Dr Clark discovered that a minute electrical charge, at a certain frequency, will kill all of the parasites without harming the body. She has developed an inexpensive device named the "Zapper" which will do this. She provides complete construction details and schematics in her book *The Cure For All Cancers*. All parts can be bought at Radio Shack. However if you are as electronically illiterate as I am, I suggest that you buy a Zapper from one of the many small

companies that supply them to the public. You may wish to call:

    a. Essence Instruments, 119 Pearl St., Kingston NY 12401, Toll Free Tel: 877-317-3341. Cost is $65.00

    b. Transformation Technologies, PO Box 2698, North Hills CA 91393, Toll Free Tel: 877-287-0712. Cost is $80.00

    c. Sota Instruments, PO Box 2698, Revelstoke BC, Canada, North America Toll Free Tel: 800-224-0242. Cost is $83.00.

3. Liver and Kidney Flushes. She also gives detailed instructions in her book on how to give yourself a liver and kidney flush. I have done these flushes on a number of occasions. They cost almost nothing, take only a day, and give only the mildest discomfort. In short, they are a breeze. You will feel in much better health after taking them.

The Book

If this parasite information is of interest to you, you definitely should take the plunge and buy the book **The Cure For All Cancers** by Dr. Hulda Clark, MD. The normal retail price is $21.95. If your local health food store does not stock the book, you can order it at .ww.amazon.com, or you may contact Spirit of Healing, 144 N. Cherry St, #7, Kernersville NC 27284, Toll Free Tel: 877-275-3196.

Other Doctor's Comments

"It is Dr. Clark's merit to have discovered the fact that parasitic burdens play a central role in cancer." -- Dr. Alan Baklayan, Orthomolecular Medicine, Munich, Germany

"We have a tremendous parasite problem right here in the United States-it's just not being identified."
-Peter Weina, Ph.D., Chief of Pathobiology, Walter Reed Army Institute of Research, 1991

"I strongly believe that every patient with disorders of immune function, including multiple allergies (especially food allergy), and patients with unexplained fatigue or with chronic bowel symptoms should be evaluated for the presence of intestinal parasites."
-Leo Galland, M.D. Townsend Letter for Doctors, 1988

"Make no mistake about it, worms are the most toxic agents in the human body. They are one of the primary underlying causes of disease and are the most basic cause of a compromised immune system."
-Hazel Parcells, D.C., N.D., Ph.D., 1974

Testimonials

Cancer Testimonial #1

On October 8, 1998, at age 55, I was diagnosed with cutaneous T Cell Lymphoma. I was given a few months to live. A bone marrow was done and a catscan was taken four days later, coincident with the commencement of chemotherapy. A week later, the results of the bone marrow and catscan indicated a more promising prognosis -- I could live another five years. Five months of chemotherapy ensued.

At the end of the chemotherapy (February), my oncologist and I were pleased with the results. Chemo was done! He would see me again in three months.

Unfortunately in mid April, the lymphoma returned. The largest tumor was removed but two more tumors grew. The doctors felt that neither chemo nor surgery would work so they decided to try radiation. In Canada, we have a waiting period to try radiation so it was booked for July.

I was terrified of having radiation and decided to pursue Hulda Clark's book, the Cure for All Cancers, which I had bought during my chemotherapy sessions. Commencing with the daily kidney cleanse tea, and then adding the parasite cleanse, I followed the regimen in her book. Three weeks later, the tumors were gone!

On July 7, I met with the radiologist as it was a consultation only. He examined me and said, you don't need radiation, you look great. He also confirmed that radiation, as it is a 'spot' treatment, would not get all the cancer, only certain tumors. He was very interested in the cleanses I was taking and researched the ingredients while I was at the hospital. His conclusion was they were doing me no harm, in fact 'wormwood' is known in medical circles to kill tumors and advised he would render a report to my oncologist. The radiologist recommended a kidney test to ensure the cleanse was not toxic to my kidneys; however, he felt the dose was too minimal to be toxic.

August 9, I saw my oncologist and after several blood and kidney tests, was told I did not need to see him again, I could expect to live a 'normal life expectancy', I was fine! We have jointly agreed to checkups every 3 months as a preventative measure. Interestingly, I showed him a bottle of the parasite cleanse and he said I was the second of his patients to show him the cleanse, the other patient had leukemia, and was doing as well as I.

October 2, I returned from two weeks, touring, hiking and exploring the Canadian Rockies. I feel great, thanks to Hulda Clark.

I realize that testimonials can be 'a dime a dozen' but having been diagnosed with what we all dread, Cancer, I decided early in my diagnosis that I had to take control of my healing and exhaust all opportunities -- dying was never on my agenda. What did I have to lose, nothing and I had my life to gain. My two daughters thought I was crazy to do the cleanse but support it wholeheartedly now. There are many of us taking the cleanse and doing well, some who have refused all 'conventional medical' treatment (chemotherapy and radiation).

I think I owe my life to Hulda Clark's parasite cleanse.

Sincerely,
CT

Cancer Testimonial #2

We just received the great news that JL is cured
of cancer! You might remember her -- she is 30
years of age and was suffering from Stage 3 brain
cancer. Chemo was failing her since there was
new growth after the chemo treatments. She has
written you and was closely following the
parasite cleanse and using the zapper. She went to
a local clinic for a body scan and she was told
that he couldn't pick up any evidence that she had
cancer. Therefore, she had her M.D. schedule a
special test in Phoenix in hopes that the medical
community would agree with the alternative
therapist. Sure enough, results just came back that
the growth of her tumor was not only retarded but
she showed no evidence of any tumor at all!
Needless to say, she and her family have received
the best Christmas present ever.

Please send our thanks to Dr. Clark. She has
touched another desperately ill person.

JG

<u>Cancer Testimonial #3</u>

I am writing to tell our my story, which is not as dramatic as some, but VERY important to me. I had just begun reading Dr. Clark's "A Cure for All Diseases" because a friend had been diagnosed with cancer. At about that same time, my mammogram showed a highly suspicious growth. My doctor recommended an immediate biopsy, but I decided to give Dr. Clark's protocol a try first. Within 3 weeks, the lump was completely gone, and there has been no trace for 2 yrs. All of this is documented in my medical records.

Just as importantly, by reading Dr. Clark's book, I became aware of things I was using and consuming that contributed to my body's workload. I am a health conscious health care provider, but there were many things I learned about even "health store products"... As a result, I have changed my life, and my health. I continue with Dr. Clark's maintenance protocol, and will do so for the rest of my life. We now make our own soaps, lotions, and shampoos. We use many

of Dr. Clark's recipes since she had supplied
alternatives to everyday products. I try to look at
everything we use and consume through Dr.
Clark's eyes.

Chapter 7. MGN-3

The development of the product known as MGN-
3 is relatively new in the field of alternative
medicine. But it has exciting promise as a cancer
fighter.

There are more than 130 subtypes of white blood
cells that make up the immune system. The most
important are the T, B, and NK cells. T and B
cells are responsible for producing antibodies and
chemical messengers (cytokines) that mobilize
the immune system for action, while NK cells
make up the body's first line of defense. The key
to optimum immune system function appears to
be not the raw number of NK cells (most people
have them in adequate numbers), but the number

and activity of the microscopic granules within each NK cell.

By encouraging the development of large numbers of highly active granules within the NK cells, MGN-3 works to "tune up" the immune system while optimizing T, B, and NK cell function.

MGN-3 is manufactured using a patented process that hydrolyzes rice bran with the enzymatic extract of shiitake mushrooms. In published studies, MGN-3 was shown to increase NK cell activity by more than 300%, B cell activity by 250% or greater, and T cell activity by 200% . This is better results than are obtained with any other vitamin, herbal or medicinal mushroom therapies.

Stimulating these immune system cells with MGN-3 gives the immune system the ammunition it needs to keep the entire body in good health.

Sources of MGN-3

1. Better Health
    International, 2025
    Oakland Ave.,
    Indiana PA 15701,
    Toll Free Tel: 800-
    772-5568. $39.95 for
    50 capsules, 250 mg.
    each.

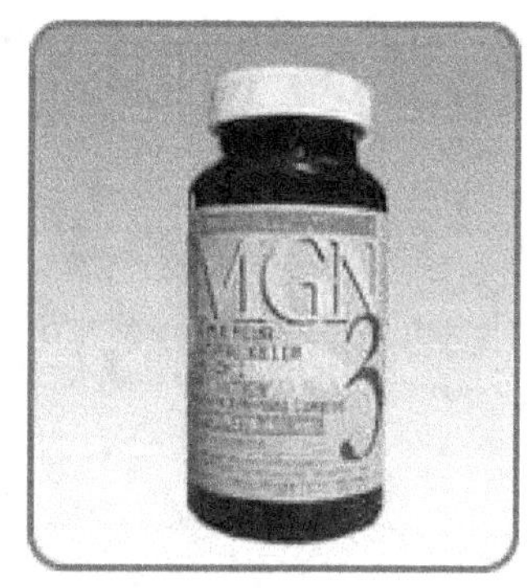

2. American Nutrition,
    5092 Buttercup Dr., Castle Rock CO
    80104, Toll Free Tel: 800-454-3724.
    $43.50 for 50 capsules, 250 mg. each.
3. Brower Enterprises, 102 S Main St.,
    Canton SD 57013, Toll Free Tel" 800-373-
    6076. $49.00 for 50 capsules, 250 mg.
    each.

> MGN-3 is now
> widely available to
> the public

Research Information About MGN-3

Following is excerpted information from several prominent research reports about MGN-3. Although a bit technical in nature, these reports are worth reviewing. Basically, they confirm that MGN-3 works!

Research Report #1

Report by: Uyemura, Koichi; Tarchiki, Ken; Ghoneurn, Mamdooh; Makinodan, Takashi; Makhijani Nalini; Yamaguchi, Dean of UCLA Medical School/Greater Los Angeles VA Healthcare System, Los Angeles CA; Drew University of Medicine and Science, Los Angeles CA and UCLA School of Medicine/Greater Los Angeles VA Healthcare System, Los Angeles CA

There is great interest among health care professionals to explore the value of naturally derived biological response modifiers to enhance immune function. MGN-3 is a biological response modifier that is an arabinoxylan compound which is a polysaccharide containing hemicellulose-b extract of rice bran, modified by enzymes from Shiitake mushrooms reported previously to be a potent immunomodulator. We have previously shown that treatment with MGN-3 had an augmentory effect on natural killer [NK] cell activity in healthy control subjects, in patients with breast cancer, and in patients infected with HIV-1. In these studies, an effect on NK cell activity was noted as early as 4 weeks and did not show hyporesponsiveness with continued treatment for over 12 months, with absence of notable side effects. In the present study, we demonstrate a direct effect of MGN-3 on tumor cell growth and cytokine production. Preliminary results showed that incubation of a breast cancer cell line (MCF-7) with MGN-3 arrested tumor cell growth, whereas control MCF-12A cells grown in a media in the absence of added MGN-3 continued to increase in cell number. Employing flow cytometry procedures, results showed that after 16 hours of treatment of MCF-7 cells with MGN-3 showed a marked stimulation in production of interleukin 10 {IL-10}. ELISA analyses of the culture media bathing the cells 16 hours after treatment with MGN-3 also showed an increase in IL-10 production, little change in INF-g concentration. However, a marked elevation in Interlukin-12 was also observed at 16 hours. **In conclusion, our findings indicate that MGN-3 acts by not only enhancing the activity of NK cells as previously reported, but also through a direct action on tumor cell production of cytokines.** The production of cytokines such as IL-10 by cancer cells to alter the activity of the immune system is well known. Our findings indicate that the biological response modifier MGN-3 can alter the production and secretion of cytokines such as IL-10 and IL-12 by cancer cells such as MCF-7; and thereby the activity of the immune system. Findings that treatment of cultures of MCF-7 cells with MGN-3 also can arrest cell growth directly may reflect an alternate mechanism of control of tumor cell growth. MGN-3, commercially known as Biobran, was provided by Daiwa Pharmaceuticals Company, Ltd. Tokyo, Japan. Work in this direction is in progress. Supported in part by VA Medical Research Funds and by funds provided by Daiwa Pharmaceuticals Company, Ltd, Tokyo, Japan

MUSHROOM AMMUNITION
© ALTERNATIVE MEDICINE DIGEST, MAY 1999

Dr. Mamdooh Ghoneum of Charles Drew University of Medicine and Science in Los Angeles compares current cancer treatment to battling terrorists. By bombing a city, you can kill most terrorists, although innocent civilians will also be killed. "Chemotherapy, radiation or surgery are the cancer-equivalents of bombing," he says, "and the beneficial white blood cells in the area are non-terrorist victims." Even after bombing, however, some terrorists may survive, as do those cancer cells that are resistant to the usual therapies. Rather than bombing the city again, however, Dr. Ghoneum advocates sending in Special Forces to locate and eliminate the remaining terrorists one by one.

Dr. Ghoneum's development of a natural supplement called MGN-3 is meant to arm the body's Natural Killer cells to seek and destroy dangerous invaders one by one. The human immune system is comprised of more than 130 subsets of white blood cells. About 15% of them are called Natural Killer (NK) cells. These provide the first line of defense for dealing with any form of invasion to the body. Each cell contains several small granules which act as 'ammunition.' When an NK cell recognizes a cancer cell, for instance, it attaches itself to the cell's outer membrane and injects these granules directly into the interior of the cell. The granules then 'explode,' destroying the cancer cell within five minutes. The killer cell then moves on to other cancer cells and repeats the process. As long as NK cells remain active, the body is able to keep disease under control.

The supplement developed by Dr. Ghoneum, called MGN-3, increases the efficacy of the NK cells. Additionally, it has other immune-boosting effects as well: it increases levels of interferon, a compound produced by the body that inhibits the replication of viruses; it increases the formation of Tumor Necrosis Factors, a group of proteins that help destroy cancer cells; and it increases the activity of T-cells and B-cells. This potent immune system booster is made of the outer shell of rice bran which has been enzymatically treated with extracts from the medicinal Shiitake mushroom. In Japan, mushroom extracts have become the leading prescription treatments for cancer. Dr. Ghoneum's findings have been demonstrated in test-tube experiments as well as seven published studies involving 72 patients. In a study presented to the American Association for Cancer Research, he reported on five patients with breast cancer. Each patient was treated with the same dosage of three grams a day of MGN-3 from a Japanese manufacturer. NK cell activity increased within two weeks and continued to do so as the study progressed. At the end of the six- to eight-month study, two of the patients were in complete remission. In a study reported the following year, 27 patients with various types of cancers including breast, cervical, prostate, leukemia and multiple myeloma were tested for NK cell activity by 51 Chromium release assay before and after only two weeks treatment with MGN-3. NK cell activity increased 154-332% for breast carcinoma, 100-275% in cervical cancer, 174-385% in prostatic cancer, 100-240% in leukemia and 100-537% in multiple myeloma.

One multiple myeloma patient was a 58-year-old man diagnosed in 1990. He underwent several months of chemotherapy following his diagnosis.

Although his condition seemed to stabilize, his blood still showed markers for multiple myeloma eight months after chemotherapy. He then began taking MGN-3 and in less than 6 months, follow-up lab work showed no indication of cancer. Today eight years after his initial diagnosis, he is the first patient known to have survived multiple myeloma, according to Dr. Ghoneum.

Dr. Warren Levin, 66, a holistic physician practicing in New York City and Ridgefield, Connecticut, had suffered from an immune deficiency with an abnormal ratio of helper cells to suppressor cells since the early '80s. "I tried herbs, healers, intravenous treatments, all sorts of stuff. Several years ago, I learned about glyconutrients — carbohydrate molecules that play a critically important role in cell-to-cell communication. I began looking for glyconutrient sources. All over the world, native populations were using substances with high glyconutrient content including Aloe Vera, astralagus, echinacea and various mushrooms. At that point, I read an article about MGN-3. I was already taking Coats Aloe Vera Concentrate together with Beta 1-3, D-glucan (Macroforce), Ambrotose, and a thymus preparation called Basic Thymic Protein A as well as the usual vitamins, minerals and antioxidants. I also did intensive mercury detoxification with DMPS. Last fall, I began

taking six capsules a day of MGN-3. At the end
of December, I sent my blood to the laboratory
and when I returned from vacation I found that
for the first time in 15 years, every one of my
tests had improved well into the middle range of
normalcy. That combination of supplements had
finally reversed my helper-cell ratio. And
normalized my mitogen/allergen responses and
NK cell activity."

Dr. Ghoneum's latest study, reported in the
International Journal of Immunotherapy,
involved 24 patients. Doctors tested NK cell
activity in each patient, administered the
recommended cancer dosage of 3 grams per day,
and tested NK cell activity again after 16 hours,
one week, one month and two months. After 16
hours NK cell activity had increased 1.3 to 1.5
times. After one week, activity had increased
eightfold. **At the end of two months, NK cells
were killing 27 times more cancer cells than
prior to taking MGN-3.**

Unlike other forms of cancer treatment, MGN-3
is a totally harmless substance and has no known
side effects. In the terrorist analogy, it doesn't kill
innocent civilians. David A. Pitts, 73, a real estate
salesman in Santa Barbara, California, had
undergone chemotherapy for lymphoma

treatments with no apparent results. "I had been getting weaker and weaker," he said. After a report on MGN-3, he sent for the supplement and began taking it while he was also placed on a course of intravenous treatment with trioxine, a relatively new drug. "In about three to four weeks on the outside, gosh, I started feeling better," says Pitts. "What really intrigued me was the idea that this supplement could enhance your immune system. When I began, I did a crash program of 14 capsules a day. Now I'm on a preventative program of four a day." At his latest CAT-scan, Pitts was in remission. "The doctor had no explanation of how or why this happened, and there's nothing I can prove. But I'm going to continue taking this for the rest of my life. What's in it is harmless and doesn't interfere with anything else."

Dr. Ghoneum has also used MGN-3 to treat hepatitis B and C and has done in vitro experiments demonstrating its action against HIV. He believes that individuals in "high risk" categories for disease can benefit from using MGN-3 preventively.

These include:
• Heavy smokers
• Heavy drinkers
• Individuals, such as artists and house painters,

who constantly work with paint
• Those born with immune deficiencies
• Families with a strong history of cancer
• Chemical and refinery workers

Research Report #3

Associate Professor and Chief of Research,
Department of Otolaryngology,
Charles D. Drew University; Research Associate,
Department of Neurobiology,
UCLA School of Medicine

Background:

Although cynicism and disillusionment with the failed "war against cancer" are widespread, I remain very optimistic that we will triumph over this seemingly invincible killer. Given the disappointing results and many drawbacks of cytotoxic therapies, it seems clear that our best hope for a decisive victory against cancer lies in immuno-augmentive therapies, those that enhance the body's innate immune response to cancer cells.

As a research immunologist, I have spent 18 years studying immunomodulating substances — natural compounds derived from mushrooms, herbs, fungi, and bacteria, as well as synthetic drugs like Interleukin-2 and Interferon. Approximately six years ago, I stumbled across a natural substance that was so promising, so profoundly superior to everything else I had ever evaluated, that I abandoned all other projects, including NIH-funded research, in order to focus entirely on this substance. The product, MGN-3 (an arabinoxylane compound), is a polysaccharide composed of the hemicellose-ß extract of rice bran, modified by enzymes from Shiitake mushrooms. As we have detailed in 7 previously published studies, involving a total of 72 human subjects, the efficacy of MGN-3 equals or surpasses the very best immune-modulating drugs available but, in stark contrast to these, exhibits a complete lack of toxicity. (Copies of complete research papers and data on MGN-3 can be obtained from Lane Labs at 201-236-9090.)

Much of the data regarding MGN-3 has been previously published in technical journals and presented at international research conferences, but the information remains largely unknown to oncologists and other health professionals dealing directly with the cancer patient. The aim of this article is to bring this research to the attention of the practicing clinician, to summarize what is known about the actions of MGN-3, and explore its present role in the treatment of cancer patients.

Anti-viral activity:

In addition to very encouraging results using MGN-3 in the treatment of malignancies, other research suggests a promising role for MGN-3 as a therapy for HIV, Hepatitis C, and other viral infections. MGN-3 has antiviral activity and also enhances the body's immune response against virally infected cells. In vitro research shows that MGN-3 inhibits replication of the HIV virus without cytotoxicity in a dose-dependent manner. Human studies suggest that MGN-3 may also be extremely useful in the treatment of Hepatitis C. In these patients liver enzymes return to normal levels within 1-8 weeks of treatment with MGN-3. The results of our ongoing clinical research into the antiviral applications of MGN-3 will be the subject of future reports.

The role of NK cells in the treatment of cancer:

Over 150 different types of white blood cells have been identified and, of these, NK cells are one of the most common, representing up to 15%

of total white blood cells. They are important because, unlike other white blood cells, they are able to work more or less independently, not requiring special instructions from the immune system in order to recognize or attack a foreign cell. For this reason, they are often considered to be the body's first line of defense against cancer and viral-infected cells. Circulating through the body by way of the blood and lymph systems, the majority of NK cells present in the body are in a resting state. NK cells become more active in response to immunoregulatory proteins called cytokines. Once activated, the NK cells become quite rapacious in their search-and-destroy activities. Upon encountering a tumor cell, the activated NK cell attaches to the membrane of the cancer cell and injects cytoplasmic granules that quickly dissolve (lyse) the target cell. In less than five minutes, the cancer cell is dead and the NK moves on to its next victim. **A single NK cell can destroy up to 27 cancer cells before it dies. Although quite small in comparison to tumor or virus cells, a single NK cell can often bind to two or more cancer cells at once.**

The absolute number of NK cells present in the blood gives little indication of the efficiency of immune function. Instead, it is the activity of the NK cells — the avidity with which they recognize and bind to tumor cells — that is important. Most immunomodulators, including MGN-3, do not increase the number or percentage of NK cells, but instead increase their level of activation. NK cell activity can be tested by means of a 4-hour radioactive-Chromium release assay. NK cells are isolated from a blood sample and are incubated in vitro with a fixed number of chromium-labeled tumor cells. After 4 hours, the percentage of tumor cells that have been killed by the NK cells is determined, and this percentage can be used to describe NK cell activity.

In a healthy immuno-competent individual, when NK cell activity is examined at an effector:target ratio of 100:1, we would expect to see NK cell activity ranging from 60-75%. However, in cancer patients, NK cell activity typically ranges from near 0% to 30%. Although it is not entirely clear whether this is a cause or result of the disease process, there is evidence suggesting that low NK cell activity may be a risk factor for malignancy or metastases, as well as a negative prognostic indicator.

Chapter 8. Summary and Conclusion

Please remember that we are researchers, and not physicians. By all means check this information out with your doctor. What is especially attractive about most of these alternative medicine remedies is that they can many times be taken along with traditional medicine protocols. So, in a way, you can perhaps have your cake and eat it too; you can follow the regimen for your cancer that is prescribed by your doctor, and you can take some of these alternative therapies also. Ask your doctor about it.

There are too many alternative holistic therapies mentioned in this book to take all at once. So you may wish to rely on your own inner guidance and select a few to try out. Generally, most people report that only a few weeks are needed in order to tell if they are being helped. You should get some sort of indication that these therapies are working. It may be a greater sense of well-being, or signs of detoxification, or signs of lessened cancer activity. Trust your inner senses and guidance.

Special Addendum

Our "Fun" addendum for Inquisitive Readers

Special Bonus Section

Do you know anyone who has skin cancer? If so, you may wish to show them this information. This inexpensive cream really works!

Our "Super Dooper" Skin Cancer Salve

There are two ingredients in our Super Dooper skin cancer salve:

Hydrogen Peroxide.

The main ingredient is liquid hydrogen peroxide. It is not just any-old drug store variety of peroxide. It is a special kind of hydrogen peroxide that is labeled **"35% Food Grade Hydrogen Peroxide"**.

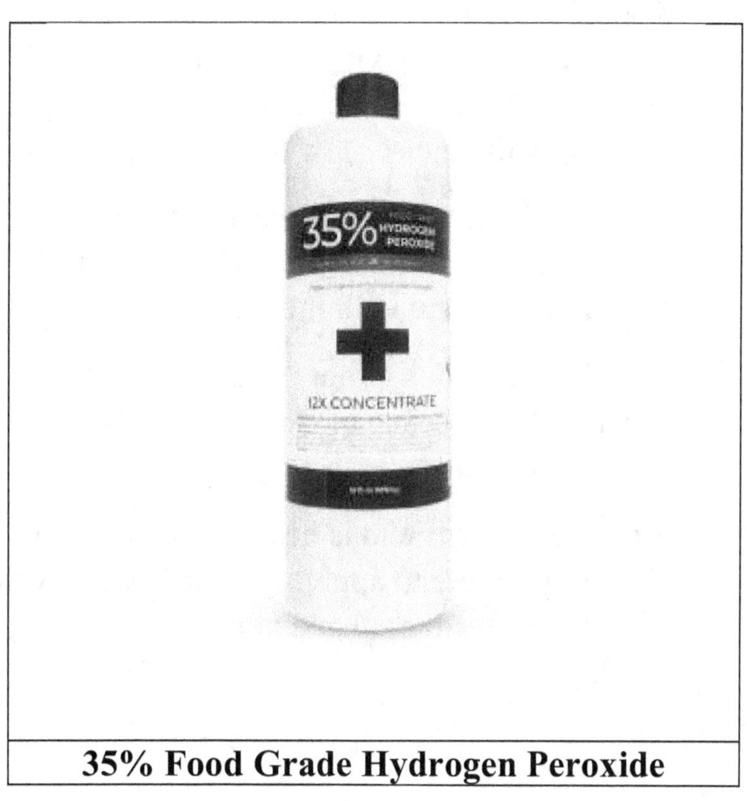

35% Food Grade Hydrogen Peroxide

This special peroxide can be found at many health food stores, or it can be bought online.

The last 16 oz. bottle that I bought cost me about $20.00. It will last me about 6 months.

How it works.

The chemical expression for hydrogen peroxide is H_2O_2. When the hydrogen peroxide is placed on your skin, it transfers to H_2O (water) and O (a free molecule of oxygen). This free molecule of oxygen is very reactive. It wants to quickly bond with something else.

If the hydrogen peroxide has been placed on a malignant tumor (such as a skin cancer tumor) it will quickly bond with the tumor.

But the cancerous tumor is anaerobic; it cannot exist in the presence of oxygen. Thus it immediately dies.

And that, dear friend is how it works. It works fast. It is simple to apply. And, in my many years of using this salve, I have never failed to see it work properly.

A few words of caution.

Hydrogen peroxide is very sensitive to light. If it is not stored in a dark place, it will deteriorate quickly. It should be kept is a light- proof bottle, and the bottle should be stored in a cool, dark place.

Also, it should be replaced every year-or-so. Age will reduce its strength.

Aloe Vera Gel.

The other ingredient is aloe vera gel.

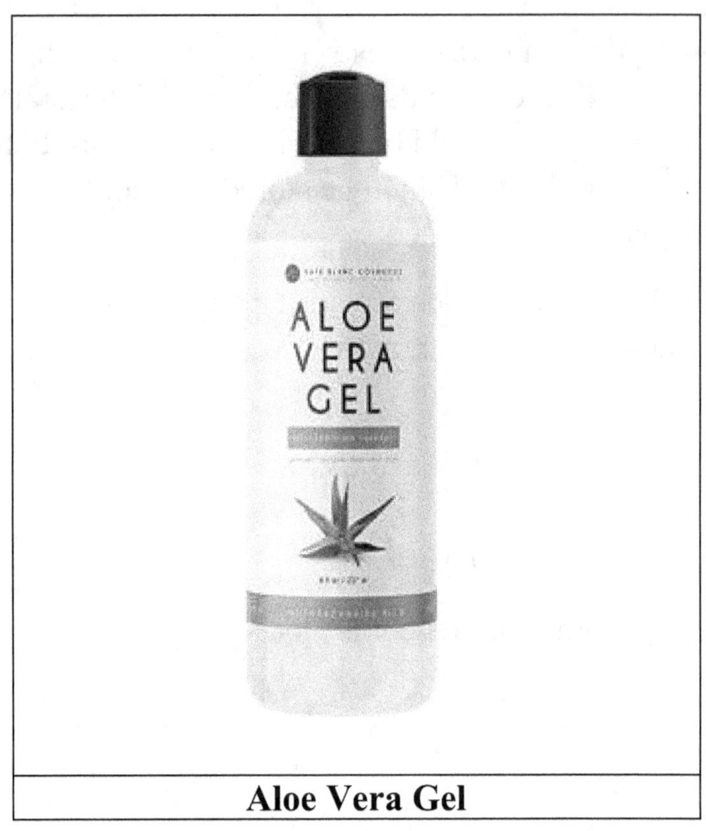

Aloe Vera Gel

This is easier to obtain. You can find it at almost any drug store, grocery store, or health food store. A 16 oz. bottle or jar costs me about $16.00.

Making the Salve:

Making the salve is incredibly easy. Just mix up the amount that you will need. Make the ration about 50% peroxide and 50% aloe vera gel. It is that simple.

You may want to use a plastic, wood or metal spoon for your mixing, as the 35% peroxide is very strong and may burn your fingers.

Store your salve in a light-proof bottle and keep in in a dark place (a refrigerator works fine).

Using the Salve:

Apply the salve to your skin cancer as needed. The more you apply, the faster it will act.

If, when you apply the salve, you see a bubbling action, this is a really good sign. The bubbling action is the active oxygen molecule in the peroxide mixing with the cancerous growth.

You should see results within a few days.

Note: This information is extracted from the book **"The Skin Cancer Information Handbook"** by Michael D. Miller.

Pyramid Power

How to shave for almost free!

My dad was an interesting guy. Raised on a farm in Minnesota during the Depression, he didn't have an opportunity to get an education. But he was smart, and had an inquiring mind. He read a lot.

So back in the 1970's he sent me a book titled "Pyramid Power". Interesting book, it elaborated on the special powers of a pyramid built with the geometric ratios of the Great Pyramid of Egypt. In the book, it stated that if you placed a shaving razor at a point 1/3 down from the apex of the pyramid, that the razor would stay sharp.

Many years later, I remembered this. So when I was experimenting with some small replicas of the Great Pyramid, I tried this experiment. It worked. For years I kept my shaving razor sharp with this method. But it was awkward because of the difficulty in keeping a pyramid structure in the vicinity of my bathroom. The smallest pyramid that I could fine to use was about 24 inches wide and 19 inches tall. There was never enough space in my bathroom to use the device. So I gradually stopped using it.

Here is what I learned: I could use an ordinary disposable razor. Normally such a razor would stay sharp for about a week, then had to be thrown away. I could place it under the apex of the pyramid. And then it lasted me for up to six months. Pretty neat. But as I mentioned, it was very inconvenient to use because of the bulky size of the pyramid.

Well friends, I have just made another discovery that I wish to share with you. I have found a very small brass pyramid that works well to keep my razor sharp. The brass pyramid is only 2 inches square, so it fits on my bathroom shelf nicely. And I bought it on the Internet for less than $10.00. I placed my razor (shown in the picture) on the apex of the pyramid as shown. I started using this disposable razor in January of this year. It is now August, and the razor is a sharp as it was on the first day I used it (maybe even sharper).

Here is a picture of my rig:

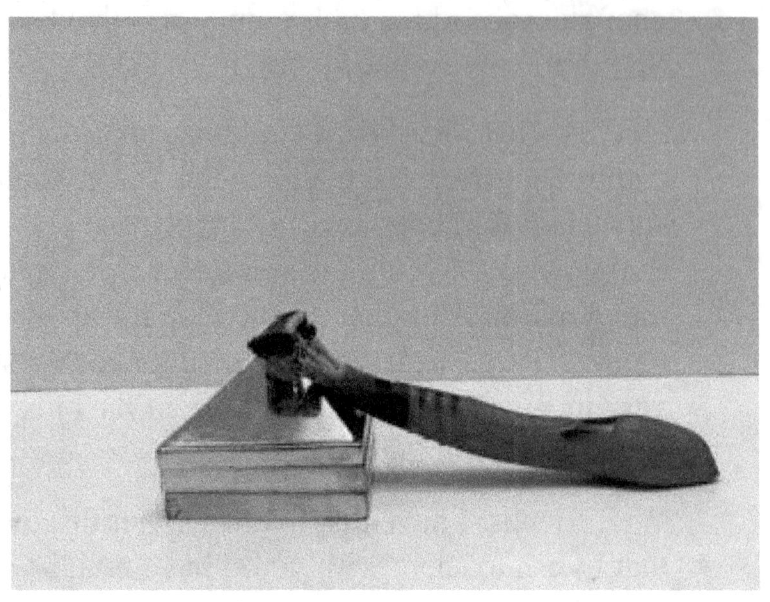

In case any of you wish to experiment with this rig, you can google "small brass pyramid". Mine came as a set of 3 pyramids. I stacked them as shown in the photo for maximum power.

As I mentioned before, the set of 3 small brass pyramids cost me around $10.00. Then the razor cost me about $3.00. If they last for a year, my total cost of shaving for the year will be $13.00. Not bad! And I still have the pyramids!

By the way, here is a list of books that I have written (some with pen names). They are available on amazon.com.

On Stormy Seas	Elk Hunting Guide
Increasing Your Cat's Life & Longevity	Kill Zone
Increasing Your Dog's Longevity	Egyptian Sacred Geometry
The Lyme Disease Handbook	Pirate History of Florida
Women's Beauty Secrets	Essiac Story and 6 Examples
Defending Against the Ambush	Two Essiac Angels
The Diabetes Handbook	Essiac Handbook
Salt and Your Health	Essiac Testimonials
Structured Water for Greater Health and Happiness	A Terrible Beauty
Greater Longevity; Rediscovering the Philosopher's Stone	Sacred Geometry
Healing Water and Cancer	Healing Water
	Male Menopause
	Women's Health Secrets
	Beating Arthritis